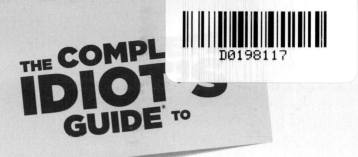

THE COMPL[ETE] IDIOT'S GUIDE® TO

Back Pain

WITHDRAWN

by Jason M. Highsmith, M.D.,
and Jovanka JoAnn Milivojevic

ALPHA

A member of Penguin Group (USA) Inc.

ALPHA BOOKS

Published by the Penguin Group

Penguin Group (USA) Inc., 375 Hudson Street, New York, New York 10014, USA

Penguin Group (Canada), 90 Eglinton Avenue East, Suite 700, Toronto, Ontario M4P 2Y3, Canada (a division of Pearson Penguin Canada Inc.)

Penguin Books Ltd., 80 Strand, London WC2R 0RL, England

Penguin Ireland, 25 St. Stephen's Green, Dublin 2, Ireland (a division of Penguin Books Ltd.)

Penguin Group (Australia), 250 Camberwell Road, Camberwell, Victoria 3124, Australia (a division of Pearson Australia Group Pty. Ltd.)

Penguin Books India Pvt. Ltd., 11 Community Centre, Panchsheel Park, New Delhi—110 017, India

Penguin Group (NZ), 67 Apollo Drive, Rosedale, North Shore, Auckland 1311, New Zealand (a division of Pearson New Zealand Ltd.)

Penguin Books (South Africa) (Pty.) Ltd., 24 Sturdee Avenue, Rosebank, Johannesburg 2196, South Africa

Penguin Books Ltd., Registered Offices: 80 Strand, London WC2R 0RL, England

Copyright © 2011 by Jason M. Highsmith and Jovanka JoAnn Milivojevic

THE COMPLETE IDIOT'S GUIDE TO and Design are registered trademarks of Penguin Group (USA) Inc.

International Standard Book Number: 978-1-61564-068-3
Library of Congress Catalog Card Number: 2010910362

13   12   11   8   7   6   5   4   3   2   1

Interpretation of the printing code: The rightmost number of the first series of numbers is the year of the book's printing; the rightmost number of the second series of numbers is the number of the book's printing. For example, a printing code of 11-1 shows that the first printing occurred in 2011.

Printed in the United States of America

Note: This publication contains the opinions and ideas of its authors. It is intended to provide helpful and informative material on the subject matter covered. It is sold with the understanding that the authors and publisher are not engaged in rendering professional services in the book. If the reader requires personal assistance or advice, a competent professional should be consulted.

The authors and publisher specifically disclaim any responsibility for any liability, loss, or risk, personal or otherwise, which is incurred as a consequence, directly or indirectly, of the use and application of any of the contents of this book.

Most Alpha books are available at special quantity discounts for bulk purchases for sales promotions, premiums, fund-raising, or educational use. Special books, or book excerpts, can also be created to fit specific needs.

For details, write: Special Markets, Alpha Books, 375 Hudson Street, New York, NY 10014.

Publisher: *Marie Butler-Knight*
Associate Publisher: *Mike Sanders*
Senior Managing Editor: *Billy Fields*
Acquisitions Editor: *Tom Stevens*
Senior Development Editor: *Phil Kitchel*
Senior Production Editor: *Janette Lynn*

Copy Editor: *Andy Saff*
Cover Designer: *Kurt Owens*
Book Designers: *William Thomas, Rebecca Batchelor*
Indexer: *Brad Herriman*
Layout: *Brian Massey*
Proofreader: *Laura Cuddell*

Contents

Introduction

This book was designed to be easy to use and easy to read. Each chapter is fairly short and chapters are grouped in four progressive parts.

You'll learn why your back hurts (so many reasons!) and discover ways to relieve your pain (lots of options there, too!). You'll find out more about your back and body that will help you communicate better with health-care providers. And speaking of communication, we'll give you the tools and wisdom to develop better relationships with your health-care providers. From acupuncturists to spine surgeons, the insights you gain will be extremely valuable in selecting the best providers for your needs.

Finally, we'll leave you with preventative care insights. Of course, exercise is a big part of back pain prevention and rehabilitation, but so is setting up your home and workplace. What you learn in the final part just might be the key to long-term back pain prevention. You'll probably wish you knew some of this before! But it's here for you now and can make your future a less painful one.

Think of this as your reference guide for back care. You could read it cover to cover, or flip to the topic that most interests you now. Either way, keep it handy. We think you'll find it a valuable resource for years to come.

How This Book Is Organized

This book was designed to inform and inspire you to know more about your body and take better care of it. We give you the tools and information in each part. Here's how we broke it down.

Part 1, Back Pain Up Close and Personal, takes you inside the world of back pain—don't worry, it won't hurt! Knowledge is power. There's no better way to get a handle on back pain than to learn how your back works and why it might be hurting. Is it a simple strain? Or something more serious? What does it mean if your nerve is pinched? Did you cause the problem or is it some genetic dysfunction?

Part 2, Relieving the Pain, will provide you with a wealth of ideas to try on your own. We take you through alternative and conventional health-care options, discuss when surgery might be appropriate, and share the promising new techniques that may be coming your way soon. Back pain is a huge problem worldwide and the good news is the medical community is constantly developing new and better ways to treat it.

In **Part 3, Meet Your Health-Care Providers,** we help you create the very best health-care team possible. As you'll soon discover in these pages, it takes a village. And with the tips and information here, you'll have the insights to create the best team. You'll know what tests may be in your future and why. You'll find out that the best doctors want you to ask questions and have second opinions. And not all doctors are alike. You'll find out how various doctors and other health-care providers are educated. You might be surprised to learn that some alternative health-care professionals study as long or longer than some conventional medical doctors.

Finally, **Part 4, Building a Better Back,** presents ideas for how you can improve your back and body every day. From exercises to on-the-job tools and techniques, this part contains a wealth of resources to help you feel better now and later. Read it, underline it, and use it!

Extras

Throughout the book, you'll see sidebars that impart valuable information in quick nuggets. Here's how they are categorized.

DEFINITIONS

These sidebars define key terms and concepts related to back pain and prevention.

WATCH YOUR BACK

The wisdom in these bits will help keep your back safer.

BODY WISE

These sidebars clue you in on how to do things correctly and what you can do to improve your health-care process.

THE BACK AND BEYOND

Here we impart bits of wisdom, facts, and myths related to backs and general health and wellness. It's all connected!

Acknowledgments

To my wife, Kacie, for her love and support in this and my many other ventures. She has immeasurable patience for the personal invasion of my career, from canceled dinner dates to middle-of-the-night phone calls.

My boys, who love to play with their "best friend," Daddy. You give me and your mother such great joy!

The SpineUniverse.com team for their commitment to this book and the spine community as a whole, both professionals and patients.

—Dr. Jason M. Highsmith

Every book is an exciting journey undertaken with many people. I'd like to thank my clients, for sharing their challenges with back issues and being willing to try new exercises and movement ideas. They inspire me daily.

Nora Tretter, my old college buddy with several back surgeries in her past, for her willingness to share her story after all these years. I admire her enduring, cheerful spirit despite chronic pain.

For help with the exercise photos: Roger Brown, Gaylon Emerzian, Rebecca Adler, and especially Rachel Herbener for producing and Dan Stevens for shooting. Also a shout-out to Jennifer Zumann of Pilates Chicago for exercise consultation, and lululemon athletica for the fab fitness clothes.

—Jovanka JoAnn Milivojevic

Trademarks

All terms mentioned in this book that are known to be or are suspected of being trademarks or service marks have been appropriately capitalized. Alpha Books and Penguin Group (USA) Inc. cannot attest to the accuracy of this information. Use of a term in this book should not be regarded as affecting the validity of any trademark or service mark.

Back Pain Up Close and Personal

Part 1 takes you inside the world of back pain. Don't worry, it won't hurt. Knowledge is power. And you're not alone: backaches plague just about everyone at some point in life. In this part, you'll learn why it's such a common ailment.

There's no better way to understand back pain than to learn how your back works. It's quite fascinating, as you'll see. Knowing a little back anatomy will help you understand *and* communicate better with health-care providers.

You'll also learn about why backs ache here. Is it a simple strain? Or something more serious? What does it mean if your nerve is pinched? Did you cause the problem or is it some genetic dysfunction? Read all about it in Part 1.

Back Talk

In This Chapter

- Why back pain is so prevalent
- Physical and psychological risk factors
- Ways to minimize and prevent back pain
- Overview of treatment options

One minute, you're going about your business, and the next, wham! Your back is out of whack. It may have happened after lifting a bag of heavy groceries or reaching for a throw pillow, or you may have simply woken up with an ache that kept getting worse. Either way, you're probably thinking, what did I do to deserve this?

Back pain is the second most common ailment in the United States. (Headaches are number one.) Back pain not only takes a bite out of your quality of life, it can grab hold of your pocketbook like a relentless pit bull. According to the National Institutes of Health, Americans spend about $50 billion every year on lower back pain, the most common back problem. It's the leading job-related disability and major contributor to missed work days.

All that may not make you feel much better, but this might: For most people, back pain goes away within a few days or, at the outside, a few weeks. You might have to tough it out for a while, but that doesn't mean grin and bear it. There are lots of ways to feel better while waiting.

Of course, sometimes it takes longer than a few days. How long should you wait? That depends on the severity and type of symptoms you're experiencing. We're here to give you some of the many reasons that back pain occurs, what you can do about it, and when you should high-tail it to a doctor.

You're in Good Company

Back pain is an equal opportunity ailment. It grips nearly everyone (men and women equally) and knows no ethnic or socioeconomic bounds. Eight out of ten adults will suffer from back pain at least once in their lives.

As we get older, we can become more susceptible to back issues, but aging by itself isn't necessarily to blame. It's how we've treated our bodies. Physical and psychological stress, extra weight, lack of exercise, or too much sudden explosive exercise can all create or exacerbate back issues. What started as a small issue can, over time, develop into a bigger deal—kind of like a crack in a dam that gets bigger.

THE BACK AND BEYOND

Most back issues tend to be from a body mechanics issue (you over-twisted that golf swing), but some occur through the march of time. Disc degeneration is associated with aging. When the cushioning discs between your vertebrae (spinal bones) begin to dry out, it reduces the amount of shock that discs can absorb. Arthritis, osteoporosis (thinning of bones), and stenosis (a narrowing of the spinal canal) are also age-related conditions.

Although some people are genetically predisposed to having back issues, most suffer because of a mechanical malfunction, such as a strained muscle. This is actually good news, because you can treat your own back in lots of ways, and when you can't, there are plenty of experts who can help.

Back pain is generally an adult issue, but children are not immune. Once again, it's more likely to be a body mechanics issue rather than one brought on by disease. We've all seen kids buckling under the weight of their backpacks. Fortunately, more and more are using the wheeled versions that they pull along behind them. That puts less stress on the back; but they should remember to switch arms, as we all should do when carrying or pulling anything.

Why Do So Many People Have Back Pain?

A number of physical risk factors can contribute to back problems:

- Heavy physical work
- Lifting and forceful movements
- Bending and twisting
- Whole-body vibration
- Static work postures

Stress and psychological issues can also contribute to back pain. How you react and approach challenges in life reflects your emotional tendencies. Do you take things day by day, or do you worry excessively when challenges come your way? How do you react if someone suddenly changes plans?

Emotions affect our biochemistry. How we think and feel plays a role in our overall well-being, and that includes our backs. Researchers have found a link between depression and back pain; sometimes back pain leads to depression and sometimes depression leads to back pain. Many times the cycle can be self-perpetuating. If you have a propensity for any of the following, you may be putting your back at risk:

- Stress
- Anxiety
- Negativity
- Depression

Behavior change is no simple feat. But catching yourself in the act might help you become aware of how you process life's challenges. Next time you're at a red light, check in with how you feel. If you find yourself feeling anxious or negative, take note of that. Be aware of situations that tend to elevate your stress, such as running late, business deadlines, or an overflowing inbox, and take steps to reduce the stress.

Risky Business

You won't be surprised to learn that people with jobs that require heavy physical labor, such as construction, are quite susceptible to back pain, especially lower back pain. It's all that heavy lifting, twisting, and pounding. But there's also plenty of kneeling, squatting, and stooping.

Bus drivers and long-haul truckers get their share of both vibration and static positions, neither of which are kind to the back over time. Repetitive movements at an assembly line may not be as intense as heavy construction jobs, but they can certainly contribute to back problems. Imagine soldering computer chips onto motherboards or stuffing DVDs into envelopes all day for hours—it's tiring just thinking about it. That's why more and more smart companies are including stretch breaks to reduce the effects of static positions and repetitive movements.

But it isn't just the blue-collar crowd. Office workers and medical professionals are also at risk. Think of surgeons, who work in static positions bending over patients; or computer techs, who are at keyboards all day. We may not be able to or want to change jobs, but some solutions can help.

Ergonomics is the term used for making environments more suitable to the way bodies move. Later in this book, we'll talk more about that. For example, you'll learn how to adjust your computer monitor and keyboard according to your body's needs. Ergonomics goes well beyond workplace issues, as you'll see.

THE BACK AND BEYOND

Repetitive stress takes a toll no matter how big or small the movement. Whether tapping away at a keyboard or laying bricks, the body ultimately needs a break. That's why wise companies, such as Netflix, a mail-order DVD business, instituted exercise breaks. It boosts productivity and reduces the incidence of repetitive stress.

Sports and Leisure

Ah, a day at the park playing soccer with the kids, a refreshing cool morning at the golf course with your buddies, or a night out salsa dancing. Life is good! At least until one of these activities seizes up your back. All involve some of the physical risk factors—the pounding of running, twisting to hit a golf ball, and rotating your hips to the latest Latin tunes. Hey, we're all about being active—studies prove it's the way to a healthy back *and* a healthy life. But preparing your body for your activity of choice with exercise will go a long way toward back health.

Professional athletes prepare. Sure, they have talent, but they work really hard to get where they are, and they have to keep doing it to stay at the top of their game. They may get injured, but they're also likely to spring back a whole lot quicker from injury because they're in such great shape. You can benefit from conditioning, preparation, and proper body mechanics, too. It will improve your golf swing and your salsa spins.

The moral is, don't fall prey to weekend-warrior syndrome: being sedentary all week, then going all out for a gonzo game of softball on Saturday. Not smart. Your body will soon scream back at you like a frantic basketball coach.

Lifestyle Choices

If you were looking for yet another reason to stop smoking, here it is. Researchers have discovered a link between smoking and the development of lower back pain. Smoking causes the proteins in the disc to break down faster. Just as heavy smoking causes changes in the elasticity and appearance of the skin, so it does to your spinal discs. That means the discs degenerate and age faster.

If you're overweight, those extra pounds stress your bones—including your spine. Your lower back and hips carry most of your body's weight. The more you can maintain a healthy weight, the better. Even if you are a healthy weight, lack of activity will impact how your back feels. Everyone needs to be active—for at least 30 minutes—most days of the week. Activity gets the blood moving and the muscles stronger. As the old saying goes, just get up and do it. You don't have to run a marathon each day, but find something you like to do that gets your heart pumping, and do it regularly.

Finally, what you eat does matter. Your whole body requires good nutrition—including your backbone. Anything that helps nourish your overall body will nourish your back. For example, calcium is essential for bones. Get it through food if you can; if you can't, supplements can help. Either way you'll need a vitamin D chaser to help your body absorb the calcium.

The Many Faces of Back Pain

Back pain can be sharp and stabbing or dull and achy. It can come and go, or it can always be there in the background, like static noise. Does it have a sensation of overall tightness, suggesting muscle strain, or does it radiate down your leg, perhaps indicating sciatica brought on by a pinched nerve in your lower back? Or maybe this scenario sounds more familiar: your back is stiff and sore in the morning along with other joints. That could suggest arthritis, a condition that inflames joints—and your spine has many joints.

BODY WISE

It's helpful to identify how intense your pain is. Health professionals often use a 1 to 10-point pain scale: 1 meaning no pain, and 10 meaning excruciatingly unbearable. Chart your pain to know whether it is lessening or getting worse through self-care or other treatments you may be receiving.

Your back is a complex structure of bones, muscles, and nerves. Any of those structures can become injured through sudden trauma or damaged by disease. The more in tune you can be with how, when, and where it hurts, the more wisely you will be able to treat it your-self and possibly prevent back pain in the future. You'll also be able to communicate your symptoms more specifically to your health-care providers.

When to Seek Medical Attention

Most back pain really will go away through time. But how long should you wait? In most cases, a few days or a few weeks will do the trick. Self-care techniques or alternative care such as massage are both reasonable as you let time help heal.

Acute vs. Chronic

Health professionals refer to pain as *acute* when it comes on suddenly and lasts less than a few weeks. Back pain is considered *chronic* if it persists for more than three months. Professional medical attention is recommended when it becomes chronic or if any movement causes severe pain.

When to Go to the ER

Occasionally, back pain may indicate a more serious medical problem. If you are experiencing any of the following along with your back pain, get immediate medical attention:

- Numbness in genital area
- Loss of bowel or bladder control
- Progressive weakness in arms or legs
- High fever that doesn't respond to fever reducers

Great Odds for Getting Better

You now know some of the good news/bad news about back pain. It may not be comforting to know that most of us will experience it, but most of us will get better fairly quickly. For those not so lucky, there are options for mitigating pain and suffering that can help with both acute and chronic back pain. Because there are many causes of back pain, not all treatments are appropriate in all cases. We detail these options later, but here's an overview of some possibilities.

Self-Care

Many do-it-yourself treatments can relieve back pain, and some things around your house right now can probably help you feel better. Heat and ice are both good choices. Ice will help reduce inflammation, and is usually recommended when pain first starts. Heat helps circulation, which can speed healing by relaxing sore muscles.

Over-the-counter medications such as aspirin and ibuprofen can help you manage pain and inflammation. Certain exercises, such as gently stretching forward, can help release tight lower back muscles, and self-massage devices are great for at-home treatments.

Conventional Medicine

Because back pain is so common, there are many experts to treat it, including those who manipulate or move your body to help release tension (generally muscular in nature). Physical therapists, massage therapists, and chiropractors all work differently, but any may be covered by health insurance.

Physicians generally work to diagnose your pain and offer prescription drugs that are often stronger than the over-the-counter variety. But you'll be surprised how many will recommend what you can buy over the counter at your local drug store. They'll also recommend which at-home treatments are best for your condition. Specialists have many options at their disposal as well, including surgery, which most will recommend as a last resort.

Integrative and Complementary Partnerships

Integrative medicine refers to medical doctors who employ both conventional and alternative medicine choices. The National Center for Complementary and Alternative Medicine at the National Institutes of Health defines it this way: "[I]ntegrative medicine combines mainstream medical therapies and *CAM* [complementary and alternative medicine] therapies for which there is some high-quality scientific evidence of safety and effectiveness."

DEFINITIONS

CAM is an acronym for complementary and alternative medicine. Complementary medicine is used in tandem with conventional care; alternative medicine is used in place of it, as when using herbal medicine to treat back pain instead of taking a synthetic drug such as aspirin.

Philosophically, integrative medicine seeks to treat the whole person: mind, body, and spirit. As such, those who practice it are more likely to recommend noninvasive techniques to address back problems, including massage and breathing exercises to manage stress, yoga to stretch and strengthen muscles, and supplements to address nutritional needs. They don't shun conventional medicine and are qualified to prescribe drugs, but most will explore other options first. Working with an integrative doctor is more a partnership among you, the doctor, and other health-care providers the doctor recommends, such as massage therapists or acupuncturists.

Alternative Choices

Anything that falls outside of conventional medicine is considered "alternative." You can explore many such treatment options with or without referral from a medical doctor; however, choose carefully and wisely. We recommend getting referrals from other health-care professionals when possible, and doing your own homework by reading the alternative section in this book to learn more about particular therapies.

Years ago, chiropractic treatments were seen as an alternative, but now it's become more of a complementary choice recommended by medical doctors and covered by some insurance. Likewise, acupuncture, a form of treatment stemming from Chinese medicine that uses very thin needles to stimulate healing, is recommended by some conventional and integrative doctors.

Different therapies work for different people. Be informed—and open-minded!

The Least You Need to Know

- Back pain affects 8 out of 10 people. In most cases, time will heal the problem.
- You can manage back pain and suffering through a wide variety of conventional and alternative treatment options.
- Some back pain requires immediate medical attention.
- There are physical and psychological factors that put you at greater risk for getting back pain.
- Lifestyle choices affect back pain. Smoking, lack of exercise, and poor diet can all create and worsen back problems.

Pain: It's Not All the Same

In This Chapter

- The biology of pain
- Map your pain and make it relevant to health-care providers
- The role of stress and psychological issues

In his famed novel *Anna Karenina*, Leo Tolstoy wrote, "Happy families are all alike; every unhappy family is unhappy in its own way." So it is with backs and back pain. When there's no pain, we're all alike in not thinking about our spines. But when we hurt, the pain is very personal and very unique.

Obviously, pain is a signal that something is wrong. But what? The causes of back pain are many and it can be quite complicated, time consuming, and difficult to diagnose. That can lead to frustration, which can certainly exacerbate your pain.

Stress. Frustration. Pain. Lack of sleep. Depression. It becomes a vicious, downward spiral. Sometimes we don't know which is worse or which came first: the pain or the frustration. The main objective, however, is to get rid of your pain. The more quickly we reduce pain, the more efficiently our bodies can heal.

Understanding more about pain in general and mapping yours specifically puts you miles ahead on the path toward healing. It guides you toward choices that are more relevant to your pain and your unique needs.

Sudden vs. Long-Lasting Pain

Back pain can come on suddenly or slowly increase in intensity over a period of hours or days. What distinguishes chronic (long-lasting) from acute (sudden, short-term) pain is duration. The intensity may be the same but acute pain will subside in time. It may take a few days or as much as a few weeks, but acute pain eventually leaves your body. Chronic pain stays.

The longer pain stays, the more damage it can do to the quality of your life and your nervous system. The experience of intense and chronic pain can make your nervous system hypersensitive, so that even small bumps, bruises, and stressors can create disproportionately troublesome pain. That's why it's especially important to nip pain in the bud.

Your attitude about your pain is an important part of the healing process. Some people let pain brew in their minds. They fixate on it; it becomes their world. They feel defeated and become depressed. When your body is spending precious resources on pain, it has less to give toward healing. Don't grin and bear it. Instead, work to reduce pain and you'll speed healing.

THE BACK AND BEYOND

According to the National Centers for Health Statistics, pain affects more than 76 million Americans. It affects more people than diabetes, heart disease, and cancer combined. Lower back pain tops the list of the most common pain, followed by migraine headaches, neck pain, and facial pain.

Where It Hurts and What It Feels Like

It hurts to sit. It hurts to stand. It hurts to walk. You can't bend over to tie your shoe or turn around without pain. And sleep? You haven't had a good night's sleep since you can't remember when. Your life is being ruled by your pain. All you want is some relief.

Getting specific about where and what it feels like will help you fight it. A numeric scale is a common tool that helps clinicians (and you) understand the severity of your pain. Again, your pain is unique to you. Be honest about what you feel. Consider such things as the intensity, sensation, and location. A chart such as the following is commonly used to help you assess your pain. A score of 10, meaning most severe pain, should be extremely debilitating. That's rare for most people.

NATIONAL INSTITUTES OF HEALTH
WARREN GRANT MAGNUSON CLINICAL CENTER

PAIN INTENSITY INSTRUMENTS
JULY 2003

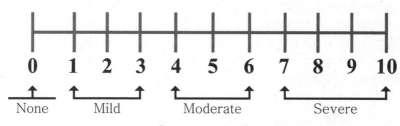

Common pain scale.

Keep a Pain Journal

Get a notebook and dedicate it to tracking your pain. If possible, keep it with you and make notes a few times a day. The more specific and more consistently you write in your journal, the better. Keep the following points in mind every time you make an entry. Like a diary, note the date of entry and the time, too.

- Note the intensity of pain on a scale of 0 to 10, 0 being no pain, 10 being excruciating. Where does your pain fall?

- What were you doing, thinking, or consuming before the pain began?

- Is the pain better or worse upon waking?

- Does activity or exercise make it better or worse?

- Describe your emotional state at the time of pain.

- Where does it hurt?

- What does it feel like? Is it tingling, burning, sharp, dull, throbbing, achy, or something else?

- What makes it better?

- What makes it worse?

This will help you determine what may be triggering pain. It will also reflect when you *don't* hurt, which can be very instructive once your treatments are under way. You'll better know what works and what doesn't and adjustments can be made accordingly.

Finally, your journal is a great place to keep health-care provider notes and contact information. Write down who is most helpful in your pain reduction journey, and take note of who isn't helpful and why. Address your concerns with them or seek care elsewhere. Either way, it will be instructive for you to evaluate them as much as they are evaluating you. More on creating healing partnerships is addressed later in this book.

The Biology of Pain

The International Association for the Study of Pain defines pain as "an unpleasant sensory and emotional experience associated with actual or potential tissue damage, or described in terms of such damage."

You know these unpleasant sensations. Stub your toe on the bedpost … a moment of silence, then comes the sensation of pain. But what is actually happening inside your body?

Nerves are spread out like a fine web throughout your body, sending and receiving messages for your brain to interpret. Pain is a protective, evolutionary asset. It causes your body to move away from things that are damaging, such as reflexively jerking your hand off a hot pan handle on the stove.

Gate Control Theory

Developed back in 1965, this theory presented one neurological basis for pain. When it comes to pain, large and small diameter nerves play starring roles. These nerves meet in an area of the spinal cord called the *dorsal horn*, where they trigger the release of chemical signals called neurotransmitters. *Transmission cells*, also known as T-cells, open the pain gate. *Inhibitory cells* keep the gate closed.

DEFINITIONS

An area of your spinal cord known as the **dorsal horn** receives sensory information, such as touch, from your body. The information is processed through two types of cells in the dorsal horn: **transmission cells** open the pain gate and allow pain signals to travel to the brain, where pain is perceived; **inhibitory cells** keep the pain gate closed and help block pain perception.

Both large and small nerve cells stimulate T-cells. But the large nerves stimulate more inhibitory cells. More activity in larger nerves, therefore, equals less pain. If the smaller nerves are more active, you will feel more pain.

Knowing how these nerves function paved the way to developing pain medications. Some reduce the inflammation that causes pain; others block the initial nerve transmission of the pain; still others may ask for more work from larger nerves, producing more inhibitory cells that keep the pain gate closed. Finally, some pain medications reduce the activity of the smaller nerves to prevent the gate from opening.

We've already talked about how the brain interprets pain signals and that the interpretation was dependent on a number of variables. It turns out that your thoughts can have a biological effect on how cells are stimulated. If, for example, you say, "Oh, stubbing my toe on the bedpost wasn't so bad," the brain sends a signal into the dorsal horn that reduces T-cell activity and that will reduce the intensity of pain.

The brain can learn to ignore some types of pain and effectively blunt its transmission. Think of the people who walk on hot coals or broken glass. That's mind over matter taken to an extreme degree.

Psychology, Stress, and Back Pain

How we think about an event can determine how our biochemistry triggers pain reactions. But can emotional stress or other psychological conditions in and of themselves cause our backs to hurt? Some health experts say yes.

Psychological issues such as the internalization of physical and sexual abuse can lead to physical pain. So can chronic stress, rage, and fear. Although pain resulting from these factors may be deemed psychosomatic, or not rooted in physical causes, the pain is very real. The same symptoms such as tenderness to touch, muscular aches, and throbbing sensations can all be felt by those who have psychosomatic back pain.

When people learn that their pain is psychosomatic, they may feel responsible, or that somehow their pain is not real. It is. And it is not helpful to cast blame. In fact, it can make matters worse by creating even more stress. Fortunately, as a society, we've begun to realize that the human experience is more than physical. Thoughts, emotions, life experiences, and spiritual aspects all contribute to our health.

> **BODY WISE**
>
> John Sarno, M.D., a physician and professor of physical medicine and rehabilitation at New York University, believes most back pain can be traced to stress. He termed stress-related back pain Tension Myositis Syndrome (TMS).
>
> Research has shown that his psychological approach to back pain relief has been effective in some cases. His treatment regime includes journaling, meditation, and psychotherapy.

Although we acknowledge that some back pain does have psychological factors as its basis, very real underlying physical conditions are usually responsible. There's no disputing that a pinched nerve causes pain.

We also advocate a holistic or whole-body approach to pain relief. The mind and body work together. How we feel influences how we think, and how we think influences how we feel. Managing and reducing pain requires both pieces of the equation.

Other Nonspine Causes of Back Pain

The reason your back hurts may not be related to your spine itself. It may be caused by some other underlying medical condition. Perhaps you have one of these conditions and may not have linked it to your back pain. Regardless, it's important to look at nonspinal causes, not only to rule them out, but to discover whether perhaps they are the cause of your pain. A doctor's diagnosis of these conditions is fairly straightforward.

- Gynecological problems

- Kidney stones

- Bladder issues

- Gastrointestinal problems such as Crohn's disease or ulcerative colitis

- Constipation

- Pain from hip problems

The Least You Need to Know

- The more you can identify the specifics of your back pain, the more likely you will be able to have it treated successfully.

- Keep a pain journal to document and track pain and treatment specifics.

- Pain has a biological basis.

- The brain can influence biochemical functions that determine severity of pain.

- Stress and psychological conditions can create back pain.

- Nonspinal medical conditions can cause back pain.

Spine Anatomy 101

In This Chapter

- The fascinating structure of bones, nerves, and muscles of your back
- How parts function separately and together
- What happens when something goes awry
- How to prevent, manage, and lessen problems

Knowing a bit about your spine and its function will help you understand why your posture and movement affect the health of your back. If something more serious is the culprit in your back pain, anatomy basics will help you better understand what's wrong. The components of your spine are your body parts. You own them for life. Why not get better acquainted?

Anatomy basics will also help you appreciate why finding the exact cause of back pain is more art than science. Sure, health professionals use many protocols and tests. But why are they poking you with a pin? Why are they asking you about your bowels and your private parts? You'll soon know.

Finally, better body knowledge will help you with preventive care and rehabilitation, and it will help you communicate more effectively with health-care professionals. So spend some time reviewing these body basics. It'll be time well spent—and just think of the new conversation starters you can throw out at the next cocktail party.

Bony Parts

Bones are efficient, sophisticated bundles of tissue, minerals, and water. Their jobs go well beyond basic skeletal framework. They are protective shells for vital organs such as the heart, the brain, and the spinal cord; they are scaffolding upon which muscles attach; and they are manufacturing centers for blood cells. Talk about multitasking! Linked by ligaments and moved by muscles, bones support a lot of weight without being crushed or broken (at least not until there is trauma or disease).

THE BACK AND BEYOND

Bones are four times stronger than concrete. The minerals calcium and phosphorus make bones (and teeth) hard and strong. Eating foods that contain these minerals, such as yogurt and spinach, helps keep your bones healthy.

Bones are living, breathing structures. They don't exactly inhale and exhale, but bones do make red (and white) blood cells. Red cells deliver oxygen, whereas the white ones rush like battlefront nurses to fight germs and diseases. If bones weren't alive, a broken bone would remain broken forever. Instead, they remarkably repair themselves (often with a little help from our medical friends). This natural ability for self-repair is the same for a broken finger as it is for a fractured backbone.

At birth, we have about 350 bones in our bodies. Some bones fuse together as we grow, including the vertebrae at the bottom of the spine, called the sacrum and tailbone. If you were a cat or a dog, your vertebral ends would form a tail able to wag happily and whip wine glasses off a coffee table. It takes about 20 years for bones to mature into an adult skeleton, which on average has 206 skeletal bones.

Bones come in many shapes and sizes, each designed for a particular function. The bones of the spine, called vertebrae, are like cylindrical building blocks. They stack on top of each other like small cans separated by little cushions called discs. The spinal column (also known as the vertebral column) is held together mainly by discs and *facet joints* with support from ligaments and muscles.

> **DEFINITIONS**
>
> The place where two bones come together is called a joint. In the spine, the joint formed at the meeting of two vertebrae is called a **facet joint.** Like joints anywhere in the body, they can swell and pinch nerves. Many people focus on the discs as a source of back pain although the facet joints are often to blame.

The Vertebral Column

The spinal column, better known as your backbone, is a strong yet flexible multipurpose structure. It holds the weight of your head and torso and allows you to move in many directions. If it were nothing but a straight, inflexible rod, we'd walk like robots from bad B-movies. Instead, the flexible spine (moved and supported by muscles) enables us to twist and hit a golf ball and bend over to tie our shoes.

The bony spinal column surrounds your spinal cord much like a conduit around an electrical cord. It protects the all-important spinal cord, a bundle of nerves that run from your brain through your spinal column and branch out to the rest of the body.

Technically speaking, the spinal column includes 34 bones. Twenty-four bones are *articulated* vertebrae bones (a singular bone is a vertebra). At the bottom of the spinal column are the remaining bones, the naturally fused vertebrae of the sacrum and coccyx (discussed later in this chapter), which join with your pelvis (hip bones). When health-care professionals refer to the spine, they're generally talking about the 24 vertebrae that form an elegant, double-S shaped line.

> **DEFINITIONS**
>
> **Articulation** refers to the motion that occurs between joints. For example, certain facet joints in the spine allow for up, down, side to side, and twisting movements.

Vertebral bones have different shapes and sizes and they get larger farther down the column. There are differences, but there are also plenty of similarities. Each vertebra has a large, cylinder-shaped body and a vertebral arch. The arch can be further subdivided into the spinous process (the bone that you can feel sticking out) and facet joints that wing out to the sides. Seen from above, a vertebra looks like a giant head with three pieces sticking out and a hole in the middle. Muscles, ligaments, and discs attach to various parts of a vertebra.

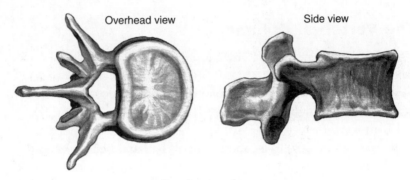

Overhead view   Side view

Lumbar vertebrae.
Used with permission. ©SpineUniverse.com.

The space between the vertebral body and the arch is the spinal canal, for your spinal cord. If this canal narrows, due to disease, for example, it can squeeze the spinal cord and cause pain. Remember, your spinal cord is a bundle of nerves and nerves carry pain signals. There are other openings among the stacked vertebrae, too. Spaces called *intervertebral foramina* are where nerve roots branch out of the spinal cord.

DEFINITIONS

Intervertebral foramina are the holes through which the nerves leave the spine. These holes are the spaces between the upper and lower vertebral bodies. The space is naturally rather narrow. If the space narrows more due to trauma, disease, or deterioration, nerves can get pinched.

Finally, let's take a look at the spinal column as a whole. When health-care professionals refer to the different parts of the spine, they reference them by the four main areas (cervical, thoracic, lumbar, and sacral). Each bone within an area has its own number. The spine is naturally curved. These curves make the spinal column stronger, help absorb shock from running and jumping, and help you maintain your balance. The size of the curves varies by individuals, but excessive curves can cause problems.

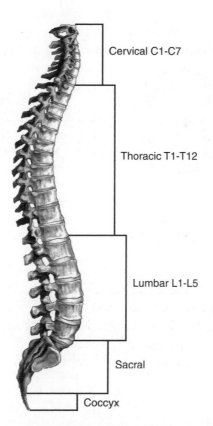

Cervical C1-C7

Thoracic T1-T12

Lumbar L1-L5

Sacral

Coccyx

Spinal column, side view.
Used with permission. ©SpineUniverse.com.

Cervical spine: This is your neck, which contains seven vertebrae (C1–C7). The last, C7 is the bone that generally sticks out the most. You can easily feel it at the base of your neck, especially when you bend your head forward. Go ahead, see if you can find it.

The cervical vertebrae's main job is to support your head. This is no small feat given that the head can weigh as much as 11 pounds! That's why how you hold your head matters so much. For many computer workers, a small but constant forward jut of the head is not uncommon. The result can transmit forces deep into the neck and shoulders. Stress to your neck muscles can lead to joint misalignment, which can pinch nerves. The result? Ouch! A sore neck with pain possibly radiating down into your arms.

Think about how many directions you can move your head. There's up, down, side to side, forward and back, and around. It can tilt like a bobble head. Thank the cervical vertebrae—in particular, the pivoting action of C1—for all those marvelous movements. And that's a good thing most of the time. On the downside, the highly flexible neck makes it especially vulnerable to injury—such as whiplash when your head is thrust forward due to impact from a rear-end auto crash.

Thoracic spine: This is your rib-cage/midback area and it has 12 vertebrae (T1–T12). Unlike your other vertebrae, these attach to your ribs. The thoracic spine can move forward relatively easily, though it's much more limited bending backward. This part of your back is not typically a huge problem when it comes to back pain (most problems occur in the lower back). The midback can, however, be overly curved in some individuals, a condition called kyphosis. It often results from bad posture—think of slouching teenagers. But it can also be caused by disease. Either way, the excessive curve makes a person appear hunchbacked.

There can be some discomfort with kyphosis caused by disease, but postural kyphosis doesn't generally cause much pain. However, excessively rounding your thoracic spine may also lead to the head being positioned forward, which, as we mentioned earlier, causes problems in your neck. The forward slumping also shortens the muscles in front of your torso and overstretches some back muscles. This can lead to discomfort when you try to sit up straight. The good news is that you can correct this with good posture and proper exercise.

Lumbar spine: Meet your lower back, the part that causes pain for the vast majority of people. But before you curse the day you were born with it, know that those five lumbar vertebrae (L1–L5) have a mighty big job to do: they support most of the weight of your body. As you can see in the illustration, being the largest of the vertebrae, they're highly qualified for the job. These bones are indeed made for walking, running, sitting, and lifting. All these activities, of course, have a potential injury risk—which you can reduce by keeping your back and abdominal muscles strong and maintaining proper flexibility throughout your back and body. Good muscle conditioning lends support to your lower back (and other parts of the spine), and with proper stretching, you can keep the area flexible as well.

An excessive curve in the lower back is called lordosis, also known as swayback. This curve puts way too much pressure on your lumbar vertebrae. Lordosis can be caused by disease, a movement of the spine such as bending the back, or bad posture. Think of the final pose of gymnasts when they dismount from the parallel bars. The chest is thrust forward, shoulders back, and the lower back arches. This is what extreme lordosis in the lower back can look like. Of course, gymnasts do it on purpose. Although it's not a disease when they perform these contortions, they can end up with back problems because of it.

For the rest of us mortals, simply sitting incorrectly can cause too much pressure on the lumbar spine. That's why knowing how your vertebrae should be aligned and taking appropriate steps to make that happen can go a long way toward relieving back issues.

Sacrum and coccyx (or tailbone): You might think that spinal fusion is something only surgeons do, but nature actually does this too and if you're over 30 years old, it's already happened to you. Your sacrum (from the Medieval Latin *os sacrum*, meaning holy bone), the flat triangular bone situated between your hips, is actually five fused vertebrae. This fusion isn't complete until you're about 25 or 30. This part is the lowest and last curve in your spine. The curve, called the lumbosacral curve, helps support body weight.

Below the sacrum is the tail end of your spine, called the coccyx or tailbone. Again, several fused vertebrae (generally 3–5) form the coccyx. Injury to this area can lead to *coccydynia*, which is a real pain in the you-know-what.

> **DEFINITIONS**
>
> **Coccydynia** is a painful condition involving swelling around your tail-bone. When the ligaments and tendons in this area become inflamed, it hurts to sit. You can also get this pain from a fracture of the coccyx, which can happen if you fall and land on your tailbone.

Joints, Part 1: Facets, Cartilage, and Synovial Fluid

The contact points between vertebrae are called facet joints. Each vertebra has joints at the top, bottom, and sides. These joints connect to the level above and the level below on each side of the spine. Their purpose is to stabilize and enable movement just like the joint in your knee or finger. *Cartilage* is the soft tissue that bridges these bone-to-bone joints.

> **DEFINITIONS**
>
> **Cartilage** is basically smooth, rubbery tissue. Your nose is composed of it, as are your ears. Cartilage caps the ends of bones, providing cushion and slipperiness, enabling bones to move easily. When cartilage wears away, bone grinds on bone, causing pain and deterioration. Osteoarthritis and rheumatoid arthritis are two common diseases that damage joint cartilage. In the spine, facet joints are covered with cartilage.
>
> **Ligaments** are strong fibrous bands that connect bone-to-bone. Their main job is to stabilize bones, holding them in place. They do, however, have a little flexibility.

Joint capsules lie between the joints. A fluid, called *synovial fluid*, is produced in the capsule. Because there is a lot of sliding at these joints, the lubricating fluid is very important in helping prevent grinding. (Cartilage also helps.) Like other joints in the body, facet joints are subject to repetitive stress injuries and degenerative diseases such as osteoarthritis. Also, the joint capsule can rupture and form cysts that pinch nerves, but most of the time, they just flare up.

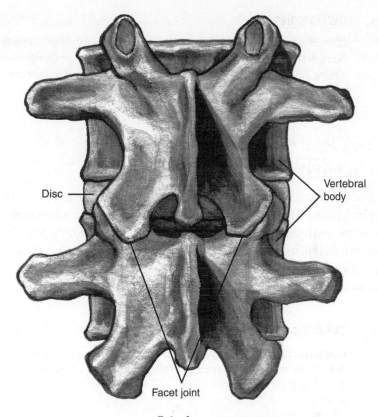

Disc

Vertebral
body

Facet joint

Spinal segment.
Used with permission. ©SpineUniverse.com.

Joints, Part 2: SI Joints

The *sacroiliac (SI) joints* link your sacrum to your pelvis, specifically to your *iliac bones.* You can easily feel your iliac bones; they're the bones at the top of your hips. Strong *ligaments* stabilize and attach your sacrum to your hip bones. Some motion is possible through these joints, but it's very limited. Pregnancy, for example, can loosen these joints, and if they don't return to normal, they can cause instability issues later in life.

The SI joint can be an overlooked source of back pain; it's subject to the same things that can happen to other joints, such as osteoarthritis. Also keep in mind the weight this lowest part of your spine bears. Excessive body weight and lifting injuries can negatively affect these joints. Because lots of muscles attach to the sacrum, muscular weakness or imbalances can misalign joints and be possible sources of pain.

Shock-Absorbing Discs

Tough on the outside with a softer, gel-like fluid inside, discs sit between each vertebra. Think of them as car tires on their sides, filled with a thick gel. When your car drives over a bump, the rubber tire 'gives' a little, to absorb the bump. Similarly, each time we move the spine, the discs change shape in relation to the movement. Like so many structures in the body, discs are multifunctional. They are shock absorbers, and they connect and protect vertebral bones. Without discs, bone would touch bone with each movement and eventually grind away.

THE BACK AND BEYOND

Discs are made from collagen; technically speaking, they are *fibrocartilage,* which means they consist of strong fibers with some elasticity.

Also know that the shocks absorbed are usually small and not a problem generally speaking, especially because these discs are quite tough. They do, however, have their limits, just like tires. When the shock is too extreme, something has to give and a tire will blow. In the case of our intervertebral discs, the gel on the inside can burst out (causing a herniated disc) or the outside can protrude (a bulging disc); the discs can also dry out and get thinner (due to disease or sometimes from aging).

Because problems can occur in either the tough outer shell or the gel inner portion, it's good to know what both look like and what your doctor is talking about.

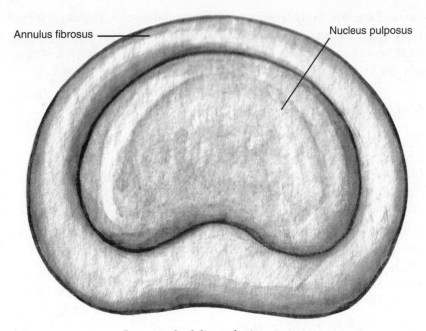

Annulus fibrosus

Nucleus pulposus

Intervertebral disc and spine segment.
Used with permission. ©SpineUniverse.com.

The outer layer of the disc is called the *annulus fibrosus*. Its main job is to attach to the vertebra above and below, although it also provides some cushion. The fibers are crisscrossed, making the connections super strong. Repetitive stress can sometimes cause this outer layer to bulge. If the bulge pushes on a nerve, the result is pain.

The *nucleus pulposus* is the gel-like center of the disc designed to absorb shock and provide lubrication. It's mostly made of water. As we age, it can dry up a bit, making the discs thinner and less shock absorbent. There is some evidence that inversion therapy or lumbar traction can help the discs rehydrate, but the long-term benefits have yet to be demonstrated.

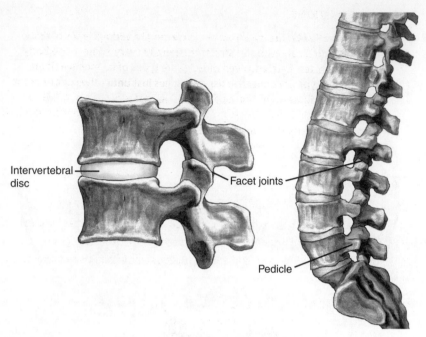

Intervertebral disc, overhead view.
Used with permission. ©SpineUniverse.com.

Stabilizers and Movers

Skeletal bones form the framework of our bodies, and in the previous section we talked about the joints and discs that link the bones. But something has to secure all these pieces in place. These are mainly ligaments, *tendons*, and muscles—all types of *connective tissue*. Each provides both stability and mobility to a greater or lesser degree.

> **DEFINITIONS**
>
> Muscles connect to bones through **tendons.** When a muscle contracts, the signal is concentrated through the tendon, which moves the bone. Tendons are firmly attached to bones. Although it isn't common, tendonitis, or inflammation of tendons, can occur even in the spine.

DEFINITIONS

Connective tissue is a broad term referring to various types of tissue that connect and support structures literally everywhere in the body. Collagen, tendons, and even muscles are types of connective tissue. Fascia, a type of connective tissue that lies just under the surface of the skin, can tighten and cause pain in various parts of the body, including the back. Some diseases such as rheumatoid arthritis are considered connective tissue disorders.

Ligaments

Ligaments are like the chief of security, whose job it is to prevent suspicious activity while allowing normal activity. Likewise, spinal ligaments allow some forward, back, and side motion, but they put on the brakes to reduce excessive motion that could cause damage.

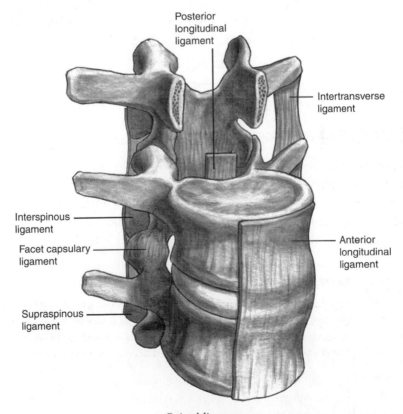

Posterior
longitudinal
ligament

Intertransverse
ligament

Interspinous
ligament

Facet capsulary
ligament

Anterior
longitudinal
ligament

Supraspinous
ligament

Spinal ligaments.
Used with permission. ©SpineUniverse.com.

Ligaments are strong, fibrous bands that have some but not much elasticity. Long ligaments secure the spinal column from the front and back; smaller ligaments attach and secure portions of the vertebra together. Specifically, the *anterior longitudinal ligament* attaches along the front of the vertebrae and limits how much we can bend backward. The *posterior longitudinal ligament* runs along the back of the vertebrae, and the *supraspinous ligament* attaches to the tips of the spinous processes. In combination, these two limit how far forward we can bend. Of course, it's possible to overstretch ligaments and— you guessed it—that can be a cause of back pain.

Muscles

There are two basic types of muscles in the body: voluntary (those we move) and involuntary (those that move on their own, such as digestive and heart muscles). Both types can get stronger and more resilient through exercise. We're going to focus on the voluntary muscles that move and support the spine. Lack of muscle strength and flexibility is a common reason for back pain.

Muscles are layered in the body. Some are deeper and others more superficial or at the surface. The deeper muscles are more stabilizing—helping to secure bones. Muscles of the hips and legs can also play a part in back problems, but we'll get into their roles in the exercise section of this book.

Your doctor may have already told you that to have a healthy back you need strong *abdominal muscles*, which help stabilize your whole torso. There are four types of abdominal muscles.

The deepest, *transversus abdominis*, hugs around your body like a corset. You can feel these muscles contract if you place your hands on your waist and cough. On the sides of your body, you have two sets of "oblique" muscles, the *internal obliques* are deeper, the *external obliques* lie closer to surface. Obliques enable you to twist and side bend.

Finally, there's *rectus abdominis*, better known as the "six pack." Although you can sculpt these into those desirable washboard abs (with a whole lot of work), they're not particularly helpful in stabilizing your back. Their main job is to pull you forward (think sit-ups and crunches). They do help you compress the deeper ab muscles, but when it comes to stabilizing the spine, you want to strengthen the deepest ab muscles, transversus and internal obliques, along with the back muscles. Among the most effective ab and back workouts are Pilates exercises, which target all abdominal and spine muscles quite well.

Deep within the body are two muscles, one on either side of the body, called the *iliopsoas muscles,* or the *psoas* (pronounced *so-as*). These are hip and thigh flexors, meaning they lift the thighs, as in going upstairs, walking. When your legs are stationary, the psoas enable you to bend forward or flex in the hips. When sitting, the psoas help stabilize you in an upright position. One of the largest and thickest muscles in the body, the psoas extend from your lumbar vertebrae, cross in front of each hip, and attach on the inside-top of the thigh bone. Sitting for long periods can constrict or shorten psoas, which can cause pain upon standing.

Like your abs, *spinal muscles* are layered. The deepest are small and attach vertebra to one another. At the deepest level, *interspinalis* muscles connect to your spinous processes; thank them for helping you stretch backward. The *transversospinalis* group forms a chevron-like pattern along the back of your spine and helps you side bend and twist, and it also assists in back bending. The next layer up is the *erector spinae.* The main job of this group is also back bending, although they also assist with side bending. Often when we get muscle spasms in the back, it's in the erector spinae muscles.

The next level consists of the *rhomboids,* between your shoulder blades, which through exercise or physical therapy can help realign your vertebrae. The very large, winglike muscles on either side of your back are called *latissmius dorsi.* In addition to stabilizing the back, these muscles help you do all kinds of things, including pull-ups. Finally, the *trapezius* muscles extend from your neck and midback to your shoulders. These muscles help you move your neck and lift your shoulder blades. When we get tense, we tend to lift our shoulders, which can make these muscles quite tight and sore.

Communications Central

All nerves ultimately connect to the brain. There are basically two major types of nerves: sensory and motor. *Sensory nerves* send information such as touch, temperature, and pain to the brain and spinal cord. *Motor nerves* send signals from the brain back into the muscles, causing them to contract either voluntarily or reflexively.

The nerves of the *peripheral nervous system (PNS)* extend down the spinal canal and branch out in 31 pairs at openings in the vertebrae called *foraminae.* They are messengers to and from your brain (or central nervous system), sending pain signals and initiating movement—like, 'Hey, take your hand off the stove, it's hot!' These nerves reflexively cause your spine to twist and turn when you walk to keep you in balance. And they keep you glued to your car seat as you turn a corner at high speeds!

> **DEFINITIONS**
>
> The **peripheral nervous system (PNS)** is the collective of the millions of nerves throughout your torso and limbs. The PNS nerves convey messages to your central nervous system (CNS), which is the brain and spinal cord.

In case you're wondering, *cranial nerves* (the ones in your head) supply the sense organs and muscles in your head.

The Spinal Cord

The spinal cord is a tubelike structure filled with a bundle of nerves and *cerebrospinal fluid,* which protects and nourishes the cord. Other protectors of the spinal cord include linings called *meninges* and vertebral bones. The spinal cord is about an inch across at its widest point and about 18 inches long.

> **DEFINITIONS**
>
> The three types of membranes that surround the spinal cord are referred to as **meninges.** From the outer layer to the innermost layer, they are dura mater, arachnoid mater, and pia mater. These membranes can sometimes be damaged by disease or trauma. Arachnoiditis is caused by an inflammation of the arachnoid lining resulting in severe stinging and burning pain. It can occur after surgery and can cause scarring of nerves.

Nerves exit the spinal column in pairs and branch out like a delicate web throughout the rest of the body. Each area of the body is controlled by specific spinal nerves. The placement is fairly logical. For example, nerves in the cervical spine (neck area) branch out into your arms, which is why sometimes a neck issue can lead to pain radiating down your arms. Nerves in the thoracic spine govern the middle of the body, those in the lumbar spine extend into the outer legs, and the sacral nerves control the middle of the legs and organ functions of the pelvis.

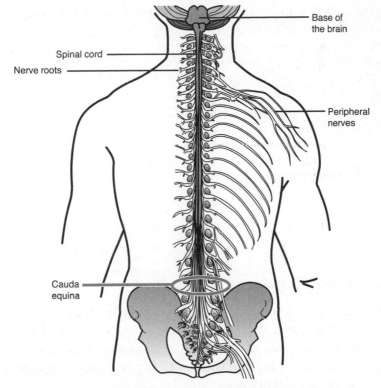

Spinal cord and nerve structures.

THE BACK AND BEYOND

When the problem is in one part of your body yet pain is felt elsewhere, health professionals call it *referred* pain.

Nerves

As we mentioned, the nerves that exit the spinal cord do so in pairs: one is a sensory nerve; the other is a motor nerve. It's probably no surprise to learn that motor nerves drive movement and bodily function. If you damage a motor nerve, you might have a weakness in a muscle or loss of function—for example, loss of bladder control. If, however, you can't feel the prick of a pin in your foot, you've lost some sensation, which indicates a problem with your sensory nerves, which govern pressure, pain, temperature, and other such sensations. This is why a doctor might gently poke you with a pin and ask about your bowel movements. If you can't feel the pin or have had a problem with bowel movements, it's a symptom of nerve damage.

A problem with a sensory nerve can sometimes feel like a sharp, electrical pain, which is why good athletic instructors will tell their students to stop if they ever feel this kind of pain. It's not a good idea to persist in any activities that result in this sensation because it could cause further nerve damage.

Cauda Equina

The spinal cord ends in the lumbar spine, where the nerves extend in a bundle of strands called *cauda equina*, so called because the mass looks like a horse tail. The nerves here provide motor and sensory function to the legs, intestines, genitals, and bladder. Suspected compression of these nerves is considered an emergency situation and requires immediate attention.

Whew! That completes our anatomy chapter. Good thing there's not a test, right? As you can see, the back is a complex network of bone, muscle, and nerves. That's why it's so hard to figure out exactly what's wrong when your back hurts. Could be a muscular issue, could be a compressed nerve, could be a misaligned vertebra—or it could be all three. At least with a little knowledge you can appreciate the complexity of the marvelous machine that your back is, and be better prepared when you visit health-care professionals.

The Least You Need to Know

- The spine is a stack of cylindrical bones called vertebrae. They form a natural double S-curve from your head to your hips.
- The SI joint formed where the sacrum and tailbone intersect with the hips and can be an overlooked source of back pain.
- Abdominal and back muscles support your spine.
- Nerves run down your spinal column and exit out to the rest of the body. Nerves can be compressed due to trauma or diseases, leading to pain and lack of organ or limb function.
- Highly intricate vertebral bones are supported by ligaments and moved by muscles.
- Intervertebral discs create a cushion between the vertebrae and also absorb the shock of movement.

Ouch! Why Backs Hurt

In This Chapter

- The most likely reason why your back hurts
- Activities that lead to back pain and what you can do about it
- Less frequent causes of back pain
- Rare causes of back pain
- The role of stress in back pain

Diagnosing back pain is as simple as diagnosing the cause of a headache—which is to say, it's not simple at all. If you read the preceding chapter on anatomy, you know the back is one complicated piece of machinery. Think about all the things that can go wrong with your computer and you can appreciate why diagnosing the human machine can be so challenging.

This chapter focuses on the many conditions and situations that can cause back pain. In many cases, the same tests and treatments may be recommended, including physical, neurological, and imaging tests. We'll cover those in detail later in the book.

In this chapter, we share with you the many reasons why your back may hurt. It's good to get acquainted with these because doing so puts you in the know. But don't fall prey to hypochondria. Statistically speaking, your back pain is most likely due to sprain or strain, the most common reasons why backs hurt.

Common Sprains and Strains

A *sprain* or *strain* is generally not a serious problem, and no one is immune from these back injuries—men, women, children, sedentary, and active alike. Like life, it just happens sometimes. The reasons why it happens are almost endless.

This doesn't mean your pain isn't real, nor that it doesn't really hurt, a lot. Health-care professionals typically refer to this as soft-tissue pain. It hurts because a muscle or ligament (soft tissues) has been injured.

> **DEFINITIONS**
>
> A **strain/sprain** injury results in a pulled, twisted, or torn muscle, tendon, or ligament. A tendon is the end of a muscle that attaches to a bone. A pulled muscle or tendon is called a strain. A ligament attaches bone to bone. When you pull a ligament, it is called a sprain.

First Steps

Sprain and strain injuries can be caused by a lift, a twist, or a sudden violent jerking motion. Accidents and falls can also result in ligament or muscle damage. Either way, you overdid something somewhere along the line—or something overdid you. Here's what strain/sprain injuries can feel like:

- Stiffness
- Tight or achy muscles
- Muscles that spasm
- Tenderness to touch
- Range of motion limited by pain

Most doctors wisely don't advocate expensive testing early in the process. Unless there is a truly compelling reason for you to undergo tests right away (say, you fell off a ladder and can't move), you should take things slowly, one step at a time.

Before they perform any major tests, medical professionals will want to know:

- Where it hurts

- How it hurts

- How much it hurts

- How long it has hurt

- What makes it better/worse

WATCH YOUR BACK

It is not uncommon for intervertebral discs to bulge a bit, especially as we age. For many people, this causes no pain at all. But because a disc bulge shows up in imaging tests, a physician might be too quick to point to that as the cause of your pain. Surgery to repair the bulge may not relieve your pain. That's why good doctors will ask many questions and perform some physical exams before moving to imaging tests.

And here are some typical scenarios that can lead to such injuries.

A Word on Whiplash

Whiplash is what happens when your neck snaps quickly back and forth, as in an auto crash. Sometimes it might take a day or two to feel the results of whiplash, because the tissue can swell over time. Symptoms include neck pain, stiffness, and limited range of motion. Headaches and dizziness might also occur. Most of these symptoms will go away in a few weeks and may only need over-the-counter medications and heat/ice treatments.

If the jolt is so severe as to displace vertebrae and/or discs, these may impinge on nerves, causing a tingling or burning feeling in the arms. Seek medical attention if this is the case.

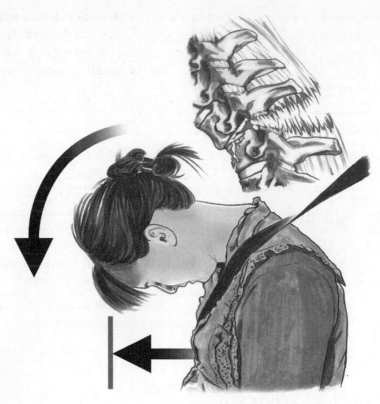

Whiplash.
Used with permission. ©SpineUniverse.com.

Deadly Lifts

Obviously, lifting weights incorrectly at the gym can cause sprains and strains. Good form when lifting objects is not just for the gym, however. Lifting heavy suitcases, boxes, or groceries incorrectly can lead to a real pain in the back, too. We'll cover more on proper lifting and exercise techniques elsewhere in the book.

A Cough or Sneeze

Like we said previously, a sudden jolt could be enough to pull your back out of whack. It's estimated that a sneeze can have a velocity of up to a 100 miles per hour. That's a lot of force! Add the likely forward head thrust and you see how even a sneeze can cause a muscle or tendon pull. It's not unheard of for a violent cough or sneeze to affect a vertebra or disc. But if that happens, the underlying structure was probably already vulnerable, and the cough or sneeze was the last straw.

Exercise and Stretching

We do have to admit that exercise has its risks, and injury, including to your back, is one of them. Usually, though, such injury results from doing too much too fast or applying bad form. Your back is especially vulnerable if you're lifting and twisting at the same time and not properly integrating your abdominals to stabilize your spine, or if you're jumping around in an aerobics class trying to keep up with a highly conditioned instructor when you're just getting started. You can overdue even a simple stretch by simply going too far.

> **BODY WISE**
>
> When it comes to exercise, the "no pain, no gain" school is out. If it hurts, you need to slow down, back off, and recheck your form.

Cutting a Rug

What could be more fun than a night out dancing? Add three-inch heels and some cocktails and—woo-hoo!—life's a party! And it just might twist or overextend your back and more.

Dancing is a great social and physical activity, but, as with all physical pursuits, it's wise to prepare to prevent injuries. If you're going to dance in high heels, practice before you go. And get some aerobic and core conditioning (recommended for men and women). All this will help reduce injury and help you look and be your best when you get your groove on.

Between the Sheets

We probably don't need to go into too much detail here when it comes to your back. It's clearly very involved in this intimate act, and it's easy to overdo it in the heat of the moment. But don't worry;

as with most strains and sprains, time heals. In the meantime, exercise other options that don't involve your back so much.

Shoveling Out

As we said previously, reaching, twisting, and lifting can be a sure-fire way to kink up your back, unless your core is strong and your form is sound. We know you want to get that snow off the walk, pronto, but guess what? You can build core strength and get the snow off your sidewalk at the same time! Lift less snow, engage your abdominals as you lift, and carefully twist and throw. This can be an awesome workout! Of course, if all else fails, hire a teenager or get a snow blower.

Pinched Nerves

The pain from pinched nerves is different from soft-tissue damage. Uncomfortable sensations might also extend into the arms (if the neck nerves are pinched) or into the buttocks or legs (if the lower back nerves are squeezed).

The causes may be numerous, but they all do the same thing: press on a nerve and cause pain. Nerves can be pinched in the spinal canal or where they exit the spine. The pain can be fleeting or constant.

Here's what a pinched nerve can feel like:

- Sharp
- Electrical
- Burning
- Tingling
- Numb
- Hot/cold

WATCH YOUR BACK

Short-term compression of nerves won't generally cause permanent damage, but the tingling and numbness can take several months to go away. If it's a recurrent or chronic issue, surgery to release the trapped nerve may be warranted.

Herniated Discs

Vertebral discs are tissues with a tough outer layer (annulus fibrosus) and softer gel-like inner layer (nucleus pulposus). The discs provide a cushion between the vertebral bones and as such are subject to wear and tear from the pressures of life, disease, trauma, or repetitive stress from physical activities.

When a disc is herniated, it bulges out and can press on nerves and cause pain. Depending on how much it is pressing on the nerve, pain may be mild or severe with a sharp or dull sensation. It is quite possible, however, that a disc bulge will not cause any pain because it is not pressing on a nerve. That's why it's really important not to rely solely on imaging tests to analyze back pain.

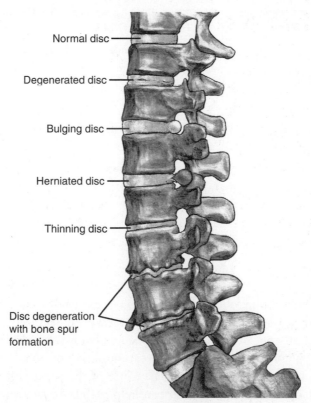

Examples of disc problems.
Used with permission. ©SpineUniverse.com.

Likewise, some discs bulge more when you bear weight on them. When you change a flat tire, the tire stops bulging when you put the car on a jack; with no weight on it, the tire (or a disc) resumes a normal shape.

If you have a bulge impinging on a nerve, treatments are generally nonsurgical and can include pain medications, physical therapy, and possibly steroids and nerve blocks. Time again tends to heal this problem and treatments will speed the healing process.

> **THE BACK AND BEYOND**
>
> Intervertebral discs do not have a blood supply to nourish them. They are actually the largest organ in the body with no blood supply. Instead, they absorb their nutrients from the surrounding bony cartilage above and below. It's a slow process, which is why it can take discs a long time to heal.

Sciatica

The sciatic nerve runs from your lumbar (lower spine) down the back of your leg to your foot. When this nerve is pinched, the pain can radiate from hip to ankle or just partially down that path. Usually, sciatica affects only one side at a time.

It can be really painful and extremely difficult to find a comfortable position with sciatica. The pain is frequently a shooting type and again can be mild or severe. It can feel worse when you bend forward or lift up your knee.

Herniated discs are frequently the source of the problem but sciatica can also be caused by other factors such as the narrowing of the spinal canal (see the following section on stenosis) or a tumor (which is rare). Most people will find relief with nonsteroidal anti-inflammatory drugs (NSAIDs) such as ibuprofen. Although acetaminophen (Tylenol) can be a great painkiller, it does nothing to reduce inflammation, which is the cause of the pain. Physical therapy and therapeutic exercises can help realign body structures and release pressure on the nerve.

Spinal Stenosis

This is a narrowing of the spinal canal or *vertebral foramen* (spaces where nerves exit). The narrowing is generally due to *bone spurs* or inflammation. As the spaces narrow, the nerves can get squeezed, which in medical parlance is referred to as compression. Some patients have a narrow spinal canal at birth and are more prone to this disease. Physicians call this short pedicle syndrome or congenital stenosis. These patients are more likely to develop nerve compression at an earlier age.

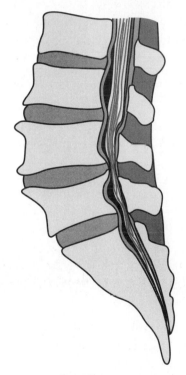

Spinal stenosis.

The root cause of most stenosis is arthritis. People over 60 years of age are especially at risk of stenosis because osteoarthritis is more common with aging. Stenosis can also, however, result from a birth defect.

Spinal stenosis mostly affects the lower back (lumbar) or neck area (cervical spine). It's rare in the middle back (thoracic). It can feel worse when you bend backward but better as you lean forward and lay down. When you bend forward, you are distracting (pulling apart) the facet joints, which relieves pressure on the underlying nerve and opens the bony canal.

Exercise, medication, steroids, or surgery may be recommended to relieve pressure from stenosis.

Sacroiliac (SI) Joint Dysfunction

The triangular bone at the end of your spine that fits into your hips (pelvis) is called the sacrum. It is a naturally fused set of three to five vertebrae. The joint between the sacrum and your pelvis is called the sacroiliac or SI joint. Problems in the SI joint can cause pain in several areas including:

- Lower back

- Buttock

- Groin

- Legs

- Pain at the top of the hip bone (iliac crest)

Pain is usually only on one side of the body. The symptoms tend to get worse in static positions such as standing, sitting, or lying down. Some people might experience more discomfort when going up the stairs or bending forward. The causes of SI joint dysfunction are many, including a sprain in the ligaments that surround the joint, muscular imbalances, abnormal walking patterns, and laxity of ligaments due to pregnancy.

To find relief in the short run, most people feel better in the fetal position, lying on their side with knees bent. A pillow between the knees helps. In the long term, physical therapy and therapeutic exercises to strengthen muscles and correct muscular imbalances can help. SI joint dysfunction can also be treated (and diagnosed) using specialized injections administered directly into the joint.

Arthritis

Arthritis is an umbrella term for inflammatory diseases that affect the musculoskeletal system. Conditions that affect one or more joints include osteoarthritis, the most common form of arthritis.

THE BACK AND BEYOND

Any word that ends with *-itis* refers to an inflammatory disease or condition. Localized conditions that affect soft tissues around the joint include tendonitis, bursitis, and myofascitis. Inflammation at the hip joint (greater trochanteric bursitis) is a common cause of hip pain often missed by focusing on the spine.

Osteoarthritis

About 20 million Americans have this form of arthritis, which can affect any joint, including those in the spine. Osteoarthritis can occur from overuse of particular joints (especially knees). The cartilage that covers the ends of bones begins to deteriorate. Bone rubs against bone, and it hurts! Symptoms also include stiffness and weakness in the arms or legs. Heat treatments, exercise, and sleeping on a firm mattress can all be helpful.

Ankylosing Spondylitis

In this type of arthritis, the joints of the spine and the sacroiliac joint inflame and stiffen. Among the first symptoms are lower back and buttock pain. In its most severe form, the vertebrae fuse together, causing a permanent bent-over position. Most people, however, have a more mild form of the disease. Only about 1 percent of the population has it and it affects more men than women.

With this disease, people feel worse upon waking or after a resting period. Treatments include medications for pain and inflammation; hot baths or showers and exercise are also helpful.

Fibromyalgia

This condition is called a syndrome, not a disease, because symptoms vary widely and an exact cause of it has yet to be found. There are no medical tests for fibromyalgia, although a link to a virus (the XMRV virus) has recently been suggested. Infections, genetics, and psychological and physical traumas have also been implicated.

It is often considered an arthritis-related condition, but it's not truly a form of arthritis because it doesn't cause inflammation or damage to the joints, muscles, or other tissues. Like arthritis, however, fibromyalgia can cause significant pain and fatigue. Also like arthritis, fibromyalgia is considered a rheumatic condition, a medical condition that impairs the joints and/or soft tissues and causes chronic pain.

There is no cure for fibromyalgia, but it isn't progressive, nor is it fatal. It is, however, generally a chronic disease, which means it persists for a long period of time. Researchers think that people with this syndrome have abnormally high levels of pain receptors, meaning their bodies chemically overreact to pain.

Fibromyalgia affects mostly women. Estimates suggest that 3 to 5 percent of U.S. women have it. They generally feel pain all over the body, although more specifically in the muscles, ligaments, and tendons. Lower back pain is quite common. Other symptoms include fatigue, headache, sensitivity to touch, and depression.

Treatments include medications to minimize pain, physical therapy, and counseling for chronic pain.

Myofascial Pain Syndrome

This is a chronic form of muscle pain that affects various parts of the body, including the back and hips. Fascia is a connective tissue that covers and connects everything in the body, including muscles. When muscle and fascia get knotted up together, the area gets tight and painful. The central point of the knot is most sensitive and is referred to as a trigger point. People with fibromyalgia often have myofascial pain.

Everyone's muscles knot up occasionally, but those who have myofascial pain syndrome experience it more frequently, severely, and persistently. Symptoms include:

- Aching muscle pain
- Muscle stiffness
- Joint stiffness
- Limited range of motion

Trigger points can be relieved through massage and a specific technique called myofascial release. Other treatments include medications and trigger point injections.

Coccydynia

The coccyx is the bone at the end of your spine, and is also known as the tailbone. As you can probably guess, the area of pain is your bottom. Coccydynia is most often the result of a fall. Sometimes people will experience pain in this area without having had a trauma event. Either way, it causes sitting to be painful. Most people with coccydynia carry around a donut-shaped pillow to make life a little more comfortable. Treatments include anti-inflammatory medications and local injections.

Fractures

Fractures are cracks or breaks in a bone. They can occur in the vertebra due to disease, overuse, or severe trauma such as car accident or fall. Fractures of the spine most commonly occur at the mid- or lower back.

Fracture symptoms include:

- Pain that persists beyond a few weeks
- Discomfort that gets worse with activity
- Pain that interrupts sleep

Fractures that severely compromise nerves include such symptoms as:

- Numbness and/or weakness in arms or legs
- Bladder, bowel, and/or genital issues
- Difficulty moving

WATCH YOUR BACK

If you suspect you have a fracture or have suffered a severe trauma, see a doctor immediately. Also do so if you experience any major nerve-related symptoms as described here.

Osteoporosis

This disease weakens bones, making them more susceptible to fractures. Osteoporosis affects women much more than men. And women tend to be most vulnerable in postmenopausal years. The disease can cause fractures in the vertebrae (and other bones, including hips and wrists).

THE BACK AND BEYOND

In anatomical terms, the front of a body or body part is called anterior and the back is posterior. Movement is described as flexion (forward), extension (backward), rotation (twisting), and lateral flexion (side bending).

Compression fractures in the spine that occur with osteoporosis are usually of the flexion (or forward) pattern. The front (*anterior*) of the vertebrae fractures whereas the back (*posterior*) does not. The vertebra loses height because it's shorter in the front than in the back. The subsequent collapse curves the spine more than usual, sometimes so much that the back appears humped. The bone collapses like a soda can and pitches forward.

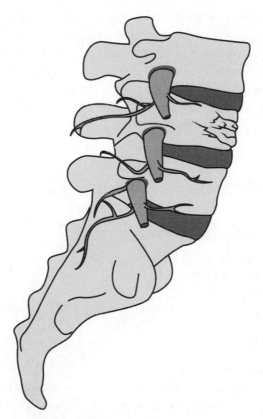

Anterior fracture in the vertebra.

Pain from factures can vary from mild to severe. In advanced cases, even simple movements can cause fractures. For example, lifting a heavy object or sneezing can cause the vertebra to crack.

Treatments include pain medications. As soon as pain is manageable, patients should walk to help keep the bones as strong as possible.

Two procedures that help stabilize fractured vertebrae are *vertebroplasty* and *kyphoplasty*. The former creates stability through injecting bone cement into the fractured area; the latter works similarly but has the added advantage of restoring height. There's more detail on these procedures in Chapter 9.

Spondylolysis and Spondylolisthesis

These two conditions frequently occur together. Spondylolysis is a vertebral stress fracture that can happen due to a birth defect, disease, trauma, or overuse. Ballet dancers and athletes in physically demanding sports that require a lot of back bending, such as gymnasts, can be vulnerable. The constant collisions in football make those athletes susceptible to spinal stress fractures, too.

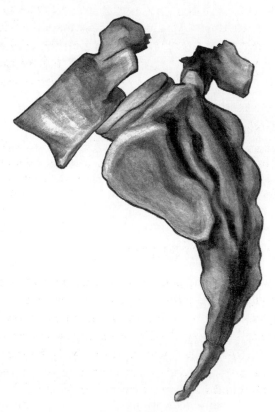

Spondylolisthesis.
Used with permission. ©SpineUniverse.com.

Once the vertebra is fractured, it can slip out of place, which is medically called spondylolisthesis. Some forms of spondylolisthesis occur without fractures, simply as a result of instability. The lower back is most likely to be affected. It can feel like a strain/sprain injury, but this injury will not get better over time. Sciatica can be triggered if the sciatic nerve gets pinched when the vertebra slips.

In addition to painkillers and anti-inflammatory medications, treatments include bracing while waiting for the body to naturally mend the bone. Building the core muscles can help stabilize this segment and act as an internal brace. If that doesn't work, surgery may be warranted.

Traumatic Injury

These injuries are generally the result of sudden, extreme force: vehicle collisions, high-impact and high-risk sports such as cliff diving or ski jumping, falls, and violent acts such as gunshot wounds and physical assaults. Fractures without pain can occur, but the bone is now vulnerable, so a less stressful impact can cause further damage.

WATCH YOUR BACK

A person who has suffered from a traumatic back injury should never be moved. The fracture could cause damage to the spinal cord, which could lead to paralysis. You should always wait for emergency personnel in these cases.

Disc Degeneration

Both traumatic events and genetics can cause discs to degenerate. More commonly, however, discs degenerate as we get older. Aging affects all tissues in the body, including the intervertebral discs. In Chapter 3, we talked about the disc as having two parts: the inner gel-like core and the thicker outer portion. Both the inner and outer parts can lose moisture and elasticity over time, which reduces their ability to cushion and stabilize intervertebral joints.

As discs shrink, they lose height, which starts a domino effect. Shorter discs cause the facet joints to change position. That leads to greater compression in the joint, causing more wear and tear on the cartilage between the bones. As this cartilage degenerates, bone spurs form at the joints. These spurs can narrow the spaces for nerves. If the nerves get pinched in the process, that's another source of back pain. Each person is different. Some people get bone spurs and never experience a problem. Others aren't so lucky.

BODY WISE

Lifestyle choices affect how our discs age. Smoking decreases the moisture in the discs. Being sedentary causes muscular imbalances, which can adversely affect discs, too. There is evidence that gentle exercise such as walking and swimming can help the discs maintain hydration.

Treatments for disc degeneration include exercise, proper body mechanics, and anti-inflammatory medications.

Scoliosis

This is an abnormal side curve of the spine. Often the vertebrae are also rotated. The disease can be genetic. In most cases, however, the cause of scoliosis is unknown (or *idiopathic*, in medical terms). It affects females more than males. And it often shows up in adolescence.

Scoliosis rarely causes back pain by itself. If there is pain, it's generally from a disc or joint issue resulting from the abnormal curve. Conversely, deteriorating vertebral discs and joints can cause scoliosis. This form of scoliosis, named degenerative scoliosis, occurs later in adult life.

Treatments vary because the degree of abnormal curvature varies. For most people, the abnormality is slight, but it's a good idea to have annual checkups to watch whether the curve is increasing. Treatments include bracing, physical therapy, and exercise. If the curve is severe enough to affect lung function, balance, or nerve function, spinal fusion is required.

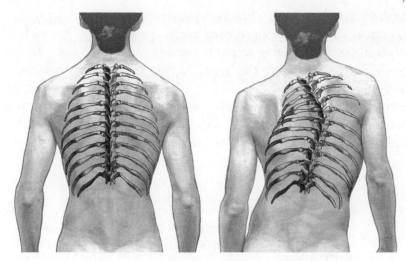

Normal side/scoliosis.
Used with permission. ©SpineUniverse.com.

Rare but Serious Spine Issues

A variety of other issues can affect your spine. Those mentioned here are quite serious. All require medical attention.

Spinal-Cord Injury

This injury damages the spinal nerves and a person can become completely or partially paralyzed. These injuries are usually the result of trauma, such as diving into a shallow pool, being in a car accident, or falling off a horse. The spinal cord can also be damaged by some of the diseases and conditions mentioned previously in this chapter. For example, the spinal canal narrowing of stenosis can severely impinge on the spinal cord and nerves.

Cauda Equina Syndrome

This rare disorder can be caused by disease or trauma. In the lumbar spine (lower back), your spinal cord transitions into the bundle of nerves called cauda equina (you remember—because it resembles a horse tail). These nerves control lower body functions including the legs, bladder, genitals, bowels, and so on. If cauda equina syndrome is suspected, emergency medical treatment is required.

Infections, Cancer, and Tumors

Infections of the spine are usually caused by bacteria or an organism from elsewhere in the body. An abscessed tooth or skin infection might be the original source. Once it reaches your spine, the affected area can become tender and swollen. Fevers accompany infections.

THE BACK AND BEYOND

If an intervertebral disc is infected, the condition is called discitis. Infections of the disc are very hard to clear because there is no blood supply to the disc.

Like infections, typically, cancers start elsewhere in the body and travel to the spine, creating tumors. The resulting pain from a spinal tumor can be similar to other back pain conditions, but unlike strain/sprain conditions, tumor-related back pain gets worse over time. Back pain that persists in a child or young adult warrants evaluation by a physician, as some childhood tumors do show up in the spine.

Psychological Stress

Some doctors believe all back pain is caused by stress. Others disagree. We think that psychological states have a very real impact on many medical conditions.

When it comes to back pain, we know there are some obvious physical causes—pinched nerves can be seen with imaging technology, as can fractured vertebrae. Follow-ups and further analysis can verify if these are the causes of pain. We also know that some pain, including back pain, has unknown physical causes. For example, muscles tense from stress. Long-term muscle tension in the jaw, for example, can cause pain known as temporomandibular joint disorder (TMJ).

Stress can cause all kinds of negative responses in the body. But what is causing the stress? Answers to these questions can most often be found through psychological counseling. This is especially helpful for those whose back pain might be a response to issues such as sexual assault, chronic illness, or depression. In some cases, back pain can be a way to deal with job dissatisfaction or to get attention from an uncaring spouse.

Of course, stress is just a part of daily living. Child-rearing, romantic relationships, financial challenges, and traffic jams can all create stress. How we react to these is an individual matter. Stress is manageable and doesn't have to cause bigger problems if we nip it in the bud. Exercise, meditation, and other relaxation techniques help a lot. We offer a number of suggestions in Part 4 of this book.

The Least You Need to Know

- Statistically speaking, your back pain is likely of the strain/sprain variety, meaning you've pulled a muscle or ligament.
- Support your sport or lifestyle activities by building core abdominal strength. Stretching can help both relieve and prevent common strains and sprains.
- Less common issues such as pinched nerves, arthritis, and fractures cause back pain and generally require medical attention.
- Aging affects all parts of the body, including the discs and bones of the spine. These can deteriorate due to disease and lifestyle choices.
- Psychological stress is a factor in back pain.

Relieving the Pain

Of course, relieving the pain is most likely the number one reason you bought this book! Part 2 provides you with a wealth of ideas to try on your own. We take you through alternative and conventional health-care options, highlight when surgery might be appropriate, and share the promising new techniques that may be coming your way soon.

Back pain is a huge problem worldwide, but the good news is the medical community is constantly developing new and better ways to treat it. They test new techniques with well-organized and relatively safe clinical trials. You can find out more about how clinical trials are conducted and whether one might be right for you.

Do-It-Yourself Relief

In This Chapter

- How heat and ice can alleviate back pain
- Over-the-counter medications—what to take and why
- Vitamins, minerals, and herbs can help you heal naturally
- Products and gadgets that soothe sore muscles
- Easing into exercise

Because most back injuries are strains/sprains, we know that they will heal with time as inflammation goes down and the ligaments, tendons, and muscles repair. Time can heal other back issues, too. Most disc herniations will naturally repair as tissues shrink, thereby no longer compressing a nerve root. But you can do a lot to help the healing process along, and that's what this chapter is all about.

Here we cover over-the-counter drugs, natural solutions, and physical treatments. Some go together well, such as exercise and pain relievers. However, if you're already taking medications for other health issues, you want to be cautious even with herbs.

THE BACK AND BEYOND

Your brain releases pain-suppressing proteins, chief among them endorphins. Natural pain-relieving methods that help you release endorphins include exercise, meditation, and laughter. So pop in your favorite comedy or read a few jokes. Laughter does double-duty by releasing endorphins and improving your attitude.

Heat and Ice

You can treat strain/sprain injuries with hot and cold packs. Both heat and ice can help reduce muscle spasms and pain, but they do have different effects. Ice reduces blood flow, thereby quieting swollen tissues. Heat, on the other hand, stimulates blood flow, bringing more nutrients to the injured site and helping to relax sore muscles.

At the first sign of an injury, start with ice to calm the swelling. Ice the area for about 15 minutes, then repeat after about an hour. After 24 to 48 hours, move to heat treatments.

Note that ice followed by heat is a general recommendation. Because both ice and heat are pain relieving, do whichever makes you feel better. There's no magic rule. Some people like to alternate hot and cold packs, whereas others prefer to stick to one temperature.

A lot of products on the market today make hot/cold back therapy easy. They can be conveniently heated in the microwave or cooled in the freezer. Look for one large enough to drape around an area. Some are specially made for the lower back and attach with Velcro, much like a weight belt.

BODY WISE

No cold pack? A bag of frozen peas can do wonders in a pinch. Whatever you do, avoid putting ice directly on your skin; it's irritating. Place ice cubes in a bag, wrap a towel around it and apply. Be patient. It takes a few minutes for the cold to come through.

Likewise, you can heat up a moistened towel in the microwave for a comforting moist heat wrap. Again, take care when applying such a wrap to your skin. You may need a second towel wrapped around the first.

Over-the-Counter Meds

Many over-the-counter (OTC) medications can help you feel better faster. Some reduce pain, some reduce inflammation, and some are combined to do both. It's important to know the differences.

Just because you can buy a drug without a prescription doesn't mean it can't be harmful when taken in excess. Some OTC meds are simply lower dosage pills than those available by prescription. Don't ignore dosage instructions. More is not necessarily better.

At the same time, know that it's easier to prevent and manage pain than it is to get rid of it. Don't wait until the pain is excruciating before you take a first or second dose. Follow the interval dosing instructions to keep pain at bay.

BODY WISE

Generally, it takes about 30 minutes for an OTC drug to take effect. For optimal pain management, pay attention to the interval dosing recommendations on the product's package.

NSAIDs: They Are Not All the Same

NSAID is an acronym for nonsteroidal anti-inflammatory drug. It describes a class of medications that reduce inflammation. They do so by blocking an enzyme, cyclooxygenase (COX). Normally, this enzyme triggers the release of prostaglandins, which cause inflammation. An NSAID prevents this from happening, inhibiting the inflammatory response.

Be aware that inflammation is the body's way of responding to injury and mobilizing cells to help repair it. However, the very same inflammation that calls for help at an injury site can also cause miserable pain. So inflammation to some degree is good. Don't worry that NSAIDs will prevent all inflammation. They most likely will just reduce the amount of it.

WATCH YOUR BACK

In addition to triggering inflammation at injury sites, prostaglandins have other functions. They regulate blood flow to the kidneys and maintain the health of your stomach lining. The downside of NSAIDs is that they inhibit a variety of prostaglandin functions, not just the inflammatory response. That's why you should not take NSAIDs for prolonged periods. Their side effects, though not common, include impaired kidney function and ulcers.

There are different types of OTC NSAIDs. All have slightly different biochemical processes but all block prostaglandins. Aspirin (acetylsalicylic acid) was the first mass-marketed NSAID. Bayer held the original patent in the late 1890s. Today you'll find many brands of aspirin. Some brands combine aspirin with other ingredients, such as caffeine and acetaminophen (described in the next section). A powdered form of aspirin (with the brand name BC Powder) is a potent combination medication that patients don't always take seriously, but should.

Note that dosages of the active ingredient can vary from 325 milligrams (mg) to 500 mg. Typically, you'll take aspirin every four to six hours.

THE BACK AND BEYOND

Aspirin, an NSAID, reduces inflammation. It also thins the blood, which is what makes it helpful for reducing heart attacks (take aspirin for this purpose only if directed by a physician). If you experience an upset stomach when taking aspirin, try the enteric-coated variety. Coated aspirin is absorbed mostly in the small intestine instead of the stomach; hence, most people can tolerate it better.

Naproxen (brand names include Aleve) is quite effective in reducing inflammation. It lasts longer than other NSAIDs. Dosage intervals are 8 to 12 hours, making it especially convenient to take first thing in the morning and later in the evening.

Ibuprofen (brand names include Advil and Motrin) is another popular OTC NSAID. Some people find it less irritating to the stomach than aspirin or naproxen. Standard dosages are 200 to 400 mg of ibuprofen every four to six hours.

Acetaminophen

Best known by its brand name, Tylenol, this drug reduces pain but has little effect on inflammation. Acetaminophen (also known as paracetamol) acts centrally on the brain and changes the way the body senses pain. Although it is less likely to upset your stomach than aspirin, acetaminophen can cause liver damage in high dosages.

It also does not thin the blood as aspirin does, which may make it a better choice for some people.

Acetaminophen is often combined with other drugs, so be sure to read labels carefully to avoid overdose. Also, because of its potential to cause liver damage, avoid alcohol when taking acetaminophen. Typical OTC dosages are 325 to 650 mg every four to six hours.

Topical Treatments

A variety of treatments applied directly to the skin can also help reduce muscle soreness and promote muscle relaxation. Some contain forms of aspirin whereas others contain natural heating sources such as peppers or plant oils. It is important to remember that the medications in these treatments are potent—so potent that they work by absorption through the skin!

The following treatments are commonly available over the counter:

- Products with ingredients such as menthol, wintergreen, or eucalyptus oil make your skin feel hot and/or cold. These can help distract the pain receptors and/or stimulate the release of endorphins. Brand names include Biofreeze, Flexall, and Icy Hot.

- Creams that contain aspirin relieve pain and reduce inflammation. Brand names include BenGay, Sportscreme, and Aspercreme.

- Creams made from capsaicin, the active ingredient in hot peppers, create a warming sensation on your skin. Brand names include Capzasin and Zostrix.

- Herbal topical formulations include those that help reduce inflammation and calm pain. Tiger Balm is the brand name of a balm made from a variety of Chinese herbs. Arnica is a popular homeopathic medicine that comes from an herb called Arnica Montana. It's reported to relieve pain, reduce inflammation, and help heal bruises. Brand names include Boiron and Arniflora.

Natural Solutions

Most pharmaceutical and OTC drugs got their start in the natural world. For example, the original source of aspirin was the bark and leaves of the willow tree. Nature-based products do heal. Respect them and take as recommended. Don't just gobble a bunch of different herbs, medicines, and vitamins. Be informed about what you're taking and why.

Herbs and vitamins don't generally have the severe side effects that conventional drugs do. It would be really hard to overdose on herbs or vitamins, but it is possible. They also may interact with each other and other medications. Ask a pharmacist, alternative health-care provider, or your doctor if you are unsure about interactions.

It's important to remember that many of these treatments are effective. They just haven't been backed by large pharmaceutical companies that spend millions of dollars on research and marketing. As a note of caution, however, they have not been subjected to the large, multicenter studies required by the Food and Drug Administration (FDA). That means they may have side effects that have not been well documented or studied. Likewise the optimal dosages, strengths, and manufacturing processes have not been established.

Vitamins and Supplements

Vitamin D with calcium is an important combination that helps keep your bones healthy and strong. It's not a pain reliever per se, but many people, especially postmenopausal women, do well to take this combination. It can help fortify bones and potentially reduce osteoporosis spine fractures. The National Institutes of Health (NIH) recommends 1,200 mg of calcium and 400 to 600 international units (IUs) of vitamin D. Higher dosages may be fine, but check with your health-care provider first.

Magnesium, on the other hand, is a mineral that can help relax muscles and reduce joint pain. This mineral supports muscle and nerve function. The recommended dietary allowance (RDA) is 270 to 400 mg for adult males and 280 to 300 mg for adult females. If you have kidney or heart problems, check with your doctor before taking this supplement.

WATCH YOUR BACK

Remember that OTC meds and herbs are still medications with some degree of toxicity. Overloading the body with vitamins or herbal remedies, or taking them in the wrong combination, may overload the existing enzymes, lead to an imbalance in chemical pathways, and even poison the body's metabolism. Remember that cyanide, arsenic, and carbon monoxide are "all natural," and each quite deadly!

Glucosamine and chondroitin sulfate supplements are a dynamic duo that has gotten a lot of attention for their potential to ease arthritic symptoms. Both substances are found in our joints and it's thought that the supplements can help refortify cartilage.

A 2006 U.S. government study, the glucosamine/chondroitin arthritis intervention trial (GAIT), found that, compared with *placebo*, the supplement provided significant pain relief for those with moderate-to-severe pain. Those with milder pain didn't seem to get much relief. More recently, two studies found no improvement with glucosamine over the long term. So the jury is still out as to the usefulness of this supplement. It may just offer short-term relief.

DEFINITIONS

Placebo generally refers to inert pills used in clinical trials. They used to be made of sugar, but then they were easily detected as such by the study participants. Now they are a safe but tasteless substance with no biochemical effect. They help researchers determine whether or not a particular substance is effective by comparing outcomes of participants taking placebo to the results of those who are not.

Another supplement getting a lot of attention for helping to relieve osteoarthritis is methylsulfonylmethane (MSM). Data from a small 12-week pilot clinical trial, published in 2006, showed that MSM was better than placebo in relieving mild-to-moderate osteoarthritis knee pain.

Fish-oil supplements contain high amounts of omega-3 fatty acids, which can help reduce inflammation. Studies have shown that fish-oil supplements may be useful in relieving tender joints and morning stiffness. Some studies say fish oil may reduce the need for NSAIDs.

Because some species of fish can contain high levels of mercury, pesticides, or polychlorinated biphenyls (PCBs), some have questioned the safety of fish-oil supplements, but fish-oil supplements don't contain these contaminants. A word of caution: In high doses, fish oil may interact with certain medicines, including blood thinners and drugs used for high blood pressure.

Herbs

Most herbal supplements for back pain are associated with reducing inflammation. U.S. studies of them are rather scant. In Europe, herbs are widely prescribed for a variety of health needs. In the United States, herbs (and supplements) aren't regulated by the government, which is why we sometimes see wild health claims about what they might cure. Choose your brands wisely by researching the brands, or ask your health-care providers for a recommendation.

THE BACK AND BEYOND

Unlike in the United States, herbal medicines are regulated as drugs in Germany. The country's health-care professionals, including medical doctors, have been prescribing herbal medicines for more than 100 years. German scientists have done a lot of research on medicinal plants. In fact, important data on chemical properties, safety, and how well the herbs work in clinical trials come from German researchers. Also, some of the most popular and reliable herbal brands sold in the United States come from Germany.

Devil's Claw is widely prescribed in Germany for arthritis, including arthritis of the spine. The herb has been used for centuries by Kalahari Desert people to treat pain. Some clinical evidence suggests it can be helpful in treating back pain.

Hyaluronic acid (HA) plays a role in tissue lubrication and cellular function. It's a naturally occurring component of the body and can be found in connective tissue, including joints and skin. The supplement is purported to support joint lubrication. Studies have been done on knee osteoarthritis, but the results were inconclusive.

Other herbs that can help ease inflammation include green tea, rosemary, holy basil, ginger, and turmeric. Again, there aren't a lot of scientific studies out there, but some of these herbs have been used for centuries in China and India to treat pain and inflammation.

Homeopathic Medicine

Homeopathy, also known as homeopathic medicine, is a holistic medical system that was developed in Germany more than 200 years ago. Its medicines are based on a "like cures like" principle. Think of homeopathic medicine as working similar to vaccines. Vaccines contain trace amounts of a disease that trigger immune responses. When the real deal comes along, our bodies can fight it.

The difference with homeopathic medicines (which are diluted minerals, plant extracts, and other naturally occurring substances) is that they are purported to stimulate the body's energetic field in order to spark healing. There's no conventional scientific evidence to support the use of homeopathic medicines. But it could very well be that the instruments to measure their effects simply don't exist yet.

Homeopathic medicines (called remedies) can commonly be found in health-food stores. The medicines are little white pills that come in small vials. They are organized by symptoms. Those recommended for muscle strain/sprain injuries include arnica, ignatia, and bryonia. Homeopathic doctors can help you choose the right remedy for your particular need.

Be Wise with Exercise

A basic rule of thumb in exercise is, if it hurts, don't do it. If a twist or forward bend makes matters worse, you need to stop. It doesn't mean you will never do these motions again; it just means you need to refrain until your back heals.

Easy Does It

As most doctors will tell you, a little rest is okay, but you shouldn't lie on your back for days on end. You need to move around, albeit carefully. Walking is a good start, as are stretches.

Your spine moves in four ways: forward, back, side to side, and rotating. You can do these movements in a chair, seated on the floor, or standing. Keep your range of motion small and make it bigger as your body allows. Again, move slowly and, if you have pain, stop.

Get in the Water

Doing exercises in a pool is a great way to get back in action. Swimming is an excellent exercise choice for your back. The water supports your body and gives you resistance, too. This buoyancy means you aren't loading your joints as much. You can walk in the shallow end of the pool, do the dog paddle, or take a water-aerobics class. If you've never exercised in a pool before, you'll be surprised how challenging the workout can be. Work at your own pace. Muscular effort is good; pain is not.

With a Little Help from Props

Wouldn't life be great if we had a massage therapist on call to ease away our daily muscle aches? Lacking that, we can do a lot to massage out our own kinks. Some handy little devices help us exercise and self-massage.

Foam Rollers

Cylindrical foam rollers are one of the best inventions in recent times. Physical therapists commonly use them with their patients with back pain. They're inexpensive (around $30) and widely available on the Internet. When you use one, you'll wonder how you did without it all these years.

Made of dense foam, these rollers come in different sizes and densities. You'll want the long version, which is three feet long with a six-inch circumference. White is the standard density—meaning it is not too hard. The gray and blue ones are usually harder and may be too hard for tender muscles. You can use a foam roller to stretch and massage back and leg muscles. Tight leg muscles can cause lower back pain.

Exercises on a foam roller include those that require you to balance, building your core muscles to provide better support for your spine. Consult with a personal trainer or see a physical therapist who specializes in back rehab to learn more about how to use a foam roller. Some illustrated books and DVDs can also help guide you.

Self-Massage Devices

There are handheld massage tools that do everything from vibrate to oscillate to thump out your muscles. Most are electronic devices, but some, such as the Thera Cane, enable you to easily press on knotted muscles with a specially shaped cane that reaches your back. Handheld devices require some effort on your part. That doesn't mean they don't work or aren't helpful, but a device that works without you having to move it (for example, lying on a roller) is the ultimate in self-massage, because it allows you to relax more.

Objects that you lie on work well for passive muscle relief. A simple tennis ball can do the trick. Place it on the floor and lie on it positioned under a sore muscle. Keeping your knees bent with your feet on the floor (rather than sitting with your legs straight out) puts less pressure on the ball. There are spiky rubber balls and those you can heat to give you an extra special touch. A wood object called a Ma Roller massages the muscles along both sides of the spine at the same time.

Chair massagers are also wonderful, although they can get pricey. A fully loaded, antigravity, body-contouring chair can set you back several grand. On the far less expensive side, there are heating pads with vibrating settings that attach to conventional chairs.

Guided Meditations

A great way to reduce the stress of back pain is through meditation. Most people do well with a little guidance. Guided meditations help you move away from the constant chatter in your head. The mind is constantly jumping from one thought to another, usually thinking about the past or fretting about the future. Sometimes we don't even realize how much static and noise we live with until we try to quiet our minds. Buddhists call the constant chatter "monkey mind."

With guided meditation, our minds have something else to focus on. The guidance can be simple breathing techniques, body-oriented work that asks us to focus and relax one body part at a time, or repetition of inspirational words. Choose whichever works for you. The key is to refocus the mind and relax the body. You might be surprised at how much better you can feel in as little as five minutes.

We offer you some step-by-step meditation and breathing techniques that will help you relax and revitalize in Chapter 16.

THE BACK AND BEYOND

There are many sources for guided meditations. Some offer free mini-sessions on the web, other have books, DVDs, and CDs. The most respected meditation teachers include Thich Nhat Hanh, Deepak Chopra, Pema Chodron, and Sally Kempton.

Back Brace

You've probably seen power weightlifters hoist more than 200 pounds over their heads wearing these large belts around their waist. The purpose of the belts is to stabilize the spine. And power lifters do well to use them, but what about the rest of us?

There is some controversy around whether or not these belts should be used in daily life. Some experts believe it gives people a false sense of security. They lift more than they are actually capable of, creating greater potential for back injury. Others say the belt helps remind people to activate their abdominal muscles before they lift.

We think it's best if you work on strengthening your core muscles and learn proper lifting technique (when lifting something from the floor, bend your knees, draw in your abdominals, then lift the object, keeping it close to your body). If a back brace encourages you to lift properly, so much the better. One really good aspect of a back brace is that it prevents you from rotating, which can minimize the potential for back injury while lifting.

Postural Aids

We put these in the same category as back braces. They can be help-ful if they remind you to use your muscles, but they're not going to help in the long run if you rely on them to fully support you.

For people who work at computers all day long, it can be helpful to wear a shoulder brace occasionally to encourage the shoulders and spine to remain in the right position. An Internet search on postural aids will help you find what's out there.

Some companies allow their employees to have a large inflatable exercise ball at their work stations. Sitting on these balls requires you to use your core muscles automatically (otherwise, you'd fall off). You wouldn't want to sit on one all day long, but if you can occasion-ally alternate from office chair to ball, you'll find it refreshing and helpful.

Antigravity Chairs

Many patients benefit from chairs that take weight off the spine. These antigravity chairs support a patient in a supine fashion, lying flat with optimal curves supporting the spine and body. It's a good idea to try one of these out before spending a lot of money on them.

Inversion Therapy

As we age and lose water content in our discs, we increase our risk of back pain from degeneration of the joints. Some patients find relief with inversion therapy. This treatment can be done at home through inversion tables. You don't have to hang completely upside down; sometimes just having your feet a few degrees above your head will help stretch your spine. There is some evidence that inver-sion can help rehydrate the discs. Certainly it can help relieve pain, but sometimes the effects are overridden the minute you stand or sit upright—after all, gravity works against you the other 23.5 hours a day!

THE BACK AND BEYOND

Although "Space Age" therapies have been touted to help back pain, a major NASA study shows that weightlessness is actually harmful to the back in the long term. Because the discs are avascular (that is, they have no blood supply), they rely on getting their nutrition from the motion of the disc across the bony endplates above and below. This does not occur in space. Thus, you lose the body's own mechanism for helping the disc heal and repair itself. With time, a weightless spine becomes devoid of nutrients.

The Least You Need to Know

- NSAIDs such as aspirin, ibuprofen, and naproxen reduce inflammation; acetaminophen does not.
- Some products combine NSAIDs with other ingredients. Read product labels and follow dosage instructions to avoid side effects and overdosing.
- Herbs and vitamins can help relieve back pain, but some may interact with other medications.
- Self-massage devices such as foam rollers and simple tennis balls can help you relieve sore muscles.
- Guided meditation is effective for reducing stress. As little as five minutes can refresh and renew.
- Use postural aids with caution. Don't depend on them to hold you up, but if they remind you to engage your muscles and foster proper posture, go for it!

Nonsurgical Conventional Medical Treatments

In This Chapter

- Physical therapy is used to help heal and maintain a healthy back
- The wide variety of prescription medications include those that can be directly injected into the site of pain
- Electrical stimulation devices can thwart back pain; some are available for home use

Back pain solutions come in many varieties, but some things are always the same: we are responsible for our bodies and our choices. What works for you may not work for me. And sometimes, finding the right medication is a trial-and-error process.

It may be easy to just turn yourself over to a professional when you're suffering, but it is in your best interest to learn about what is being recommended to you. It will help you (and your doctor) determine whether a medicine or treatment is working as intended.

Because this chapter is on conventional medical approaches, you can trust that these treatments have science to back up their claims. That doesn't mean they all work perfectly for everyone, but they've been tested over time using accepted medical standards and proven effective for the majority of people in a study. Experienced doctors have seen them work for other patients and so may be recommending them to you.

Physical Therapy

The beauty of physical therapy is it is customized around your specific body's needs. It may take just a few appointments or many sessions to get you back on track. It all depends on your unique situation and progress. A session may last 20 minutes or an hour. Fortunately, insurance commonly covers doctor-prescribed physical therapy.

The most important thing about physical therapy is that it shouldn't end when you walk out the door. Practice daily the exercises the therapists teach you and you will gain the most benefit. Also, give the exercises a couple of weeks. You won't feel better right away, and you might even feel worse for a few days until your muscles adjust to their new marching orders.

Patients are typically referred to physical therapy (also called physiotherapy) by a medical doctor. A physical therapist is educated in anatomy, body mechanics, and movement. The role of a physical therapist is to get you moving as normally as possible as soon as possible. Principles of effective physical therapy include education, therapeutic exercise, and hands-on treatment.

BODY WISE

Wear loose clothing to your physical therapy appointment. The therapist will evaluate your posture, flexibility, and movement, so you want clothes that allow you to move freely. A physical therapist may also touch you in much the way a massage therapist and chiropractor (an expert in spine manipulation) does.

Education

How you sit, stand, and walk all contribute to the health of your spine. During physical therapy, you'll learn proper movement and proper body alignment. Work and daily life often require unique movements such as picking up children or sitting at a computer all day. Learning good postural habits for all your daily activities will go a long way toward rehabilitating and maintaining a healthy back.

Often, this may require some *neuromuscular reeducation*, because the way you use your body now may be contributing to your back problems. Sure, you've been walking, sitting, standing, and lifting since you were two years old, but you may have picked up some bad habits along the way.

> **BODY WISE**
>
> To have a happy, pain-free body, we need strong, flexible muscles. Stretching is an important part of an exercise program. When muscles are too tight, they can be painful and pull our bones out of alignment. Tight hamstrings (muscles on the back of your thigh) and hip flexors (muscles that pull your thigh up) are culprits in lower back pain. It's wise to keep these muscles limber.

Exercises that address neuromuscular reeducation generally involve balance, coordination, and posture. For example, therapists may have you do such exercises as standing on one leg or stabilizing one body part while moving another, a hallmark of Pilates. Through time, you'll shed bad habits and create healthier movement patterns.

> **DEFINITIONS**
>
> Muscles and nerves work together to create movement. Over time, we develop habitual patterns of movement (some good, some not). These are stored in our muscle memory. When there are repetitive poor patterns, trauma, or damage to nerves or muscles, we may need to relearn movements or learn how to do them correctly, a process called **neuromuscular reeducation.**

Therapeutic Exercise

Many people with back problems, especially those who have chronic pain, may be deconditioned, meaning that their muscles aren't as strong as they need to be to support their bodies and daily movements. That's why exercise is a foundational aspect of physical therapy. Expect to move and be moved in physical therapy. And expect to get customized exercises as homework. Many of these will address activities of daily living—meaning proper form for getting in and out the car, walking, sleeping, and so on.

The more you participate in your recovery the faster your recovery will be. Physical therapy may include exercises with equipment such as large inflatable balls, hand weights, and treadmills.

Hands-On Treatments

In addition to exercises, physical therapy also includes various hands-on techniques (often called modalities) done in the therapist's office. These include hot/cold pack treatments, soft-tissue massage to release muscular tension, and physical manipulations that help realign the spine. Sometimes you will resist against the gentle force of the therapists' hands and other times you will be passive as the therapist pulls on a body part or presses on a tight muscle.

Physical therapy can be physically challenging and sometimes a bit uncomfortable. It'll be worth it, though. You'll be rewarded with a body that moves better and feels better. And you'll know how to keep it that way.

Prescription Medications

When it comes to prescription meds, you definitely want to be an informed consumer. Different drugs have different purposes. Some work solely on pain or on inflammation, whereas some are combined. Some prescription drugs are simply stronger versions of over-the-counter (OTC) medication. Don't mix OTC meds with prescriptions unless your doctor tells you to. Ditto regarding supplements. Be up front with your doc about everything you're taking. Some drugs and supplements may be fine taken simultaneously; others may cause unwanted reactions.

WATCH YOUR BACK

As with all drugs, take special note of whether to take your prescription with food or on an empty stomach, or whether you should avoid certain foods. Pharmacists should also be able to consult with you about any special precautions on your meds. Some medications, especially pain medicines, should not be taken while driving. You can actually be arrested for driving under the influence of some prescription medications.

Generally, there are three different meds prescribed for back problems: pain medications, anti-inflammatory drugs, and muscle relaxants. Occasionally, neuropathic pain medications are used to treat nerve pain, as are antidepressants and anticonvulsants.

Pain Meds

The World Health Organization defined a method of controlling pain known as the pain ladder. The idea is to start treatment at the bottom rung with over-the-counter drugs and move up the ladder if pain persists. If you've gotten a prescription for pain medications, that usually means you've already tried over-the-counter drugs such as aspirin or acetaminophen and they haven't worked well enough.

In the pain meds category the most powerful drugs are *opioids* (opiates). Opioids (formerly known as narcotics) are a class of drugs that includes morphine and codeine. They work well to reduce pain but carry the potential for tolerance and addiction. The stronger they are, the greater the potential. Still, they do have their place for a limited time.

DEFINITIONS

Morphine, codeine, opium, and heroin are examples of **opioids,** drugs derived from the opium poppy. The human body produces endorphins in response to pain. Drugs made from opiates can stimulate endorphin receptors. They mimic the body's natural painkilling abilities.

Tolerance is the buildup of resistance to the effects of opioids. In other words, your body's metabolism breaks down the current dosage quicker and you need more to get an effect. This is different from addiction but related. Patients develop a tolerance when the current dosage no longer gives them pain relief and they need more. Addiction occurs when there are adaptive changes in the brain leading to uncontrollable craving for a substance.

You'll probably get a prescription for codeine or a semisynthetic relative (oxycodone or hydrocodone). The following brand-name pharmaceuticals are combined with other drugs. The combination helps reduce the amount of opioids needed. These are commonly prescribed for back pain:

- Tylenol 3 (codeine with acetaminophen)

- Vicodin (hydrocodone with acetaminophen)

- Percodan (oxycodone with aspirin)

- Percocet (oxycodone with acetaminophen)

There are also stronger pain medications, typically prescribed after surgery, after a severe injury, or for especially stubborn pain:

- Fentanyl patch (synthetic drug many times more potent than morphine)

- OxyContin (long-acting oxycodone)

- Dilaudid (hydromorphone)

Common side effects of opioids include sleepiness, lightheadedness, and constipation.

 WATCH YOUR BACK

If your pain progresses to the point you need surgery, you are better off being on as little narcotics as possible before the operation. When you have tolerance to narcotics, surgical pain can be very difficult to control.

Anti-Inflammatory Meds

Prescription anti-inflammatory drugs typically prescribed for back pain are nonsteroidal anti-inflammatory drugs (NSAIDs). They work just like the over-the-counter variety in that they reduce inflammation by reducing prostaglandin production (chemicals that do many things, including promoting inflammation and protecting stomach lining). These drugs do carry side effects; an upset stomach is the most common. Your prescription is likely a higher dosage of what is available on the market.

A relatively new class of NSAIDs called COX-2 inhibitors has the benefit of bringing down inflammation without causing gastrointestinal problems. Two of these drugs (Vioxx and Bextra) were taken off the market because long-term use was linked to increased risk of heart attack and stroke. The only COX-2 inhibitor currently available in the United States has the brand name Celebrex.

Generally, NSAIDs work pretty quickly, within a half-hour or so. They are prescribed for a variety of back conditions, including arthritis and strain/sprain injuries.

WATCH YOUR BACK

Steroids are very powerful anti-inflammatory drugs. They can be prescribed for back pain but most doctors prefer NSAIDs to avoid the side effects of steroids. Long-term use of steroids can lead to weight gain, stomach ulcers, osteoporosis, and other problems. They may also raise blood sugar in diabetic patients. If steroids are prescribed, they are generally for short-term use—for example, one to two weeks.

Muscle Relaxants

When muscle spasms are causing excessive pain, your doctor may prescribe a muscle relaxer. They are a class of drug with a number of different chemical combinations. Because they have no effect on inflammation, it may be recommended that you take both a muscle relaxant and an anti-inflammatory drug.

Muscle relaxants don't affect your muscles per se; they work on your brain and spinal cord by reducing motor activity, which in turn reduces muscle spasm. In fact, they relax the whole body. A reduction in muscle spasm can be useful before doing therapeutic exercises as it allows you to gain greater range of motion. Unfortunately, these drugs can also make you sleepy. Commonly prescribed muscle relaxants include:

- Soma, which is usually taken on a short-term basis due to its habit-forming potential

- Valium, another short-term drug with the potential to interrupt sleep cycles

- Flexeril, which can be prescribed for longer periods of time

Neuropathic Pain Agents

Finally, some people with chronic pain may actually be prescribed antidepressants or anticonvulsants. The former calms down the nervous system and increases biochemicals that reduce pain signals. Anticonvulsants also interfere with nerve communication, suppressing the nervous system and thereby blocking pain. These drugs all help relieve *neuropathic pain* and may also be prescribed for other conditions.

DEFINITIONS

Neuropathic pain is nerve-based pain that reflects trauma, irritation, or chronic changes in nerves. This is different from nociceptive pain, which originates from the other tissues in the body (muscle, disc, and bone) and is transmitted by the nerves. Neuropathic agents are more effective against nerve-related pain.

It's not uncommon for pharmaceutical drugs to have more than one indication, or condition that it treats. Drug companies generally promote the drug for the indication that reaches the largest group of patients. For example, the drug with the brand name Lyrica (pregabalin) is often prescribed for people with neuropathic pain of diabetes; the drug with the brand name Neurontin (gabapentin) was originally developed for epileptic seizures. Both these drugs act on the central nervous system. Because of that, they can be prescribed for other indications, such as back pain caused by nerve damage.

Injections

Remember the pain ladder? We're on a higher rung, now. Doctors recommend injections when other medications have not worked. Injections deliver medicine directly to the source of pain. This makes them highly effective. Also, the medication tends to stay in one place (compared to oral medicines that must go through several body systems before reaching the site of pain). But we're talking about sticking needles in your body, so it is a more aggressive and invasive procedure. The skill of the specialist is crucial here because he or she needs to target the precise point in the nervous or musculoskeletal system.

Injections are generally outpatient procedures. Specialists such as radiologists, anesthesiologists, pain physicians, physiatrists, or neuro-surgeons will typically administer the shot. There are different medications as well as different points of administration. Also under-stand that injections are not meant to be stand-alone procedures; rather they should be part of an overall treatment plan that includes physical therapy. The following subsections describe some of the more common injection treatments.

Trigger-Point Injections

You know you have a muscular trigger point because you can feel it quite easily. Press on one of these knotted up muscles and it hurts there and also radiates out to other parts on your back. Hence the name "trigger," because they produce pain elsewhere.

The first course of treatment for trigger points is massage or other hands-on techniques. If they're still painful after a few weeks of that treatment, an injection may be recommended. A local anesthetic, saline solution, or Botox may be injected to relieve that muscle knot. More than three injections into the same trigger point is not recom-mended because it can permanently damage the muscle.

Facet Injections

Okay, class: Remember those joints between your vertebrae we dis-cussed in Chapter 3? As you may recall, they're called facet joints. Like other joints in the body, they are subject to wear and tear and diseases such as osteoarthritis that cause inflammation and thus pain. The medicine injected into a facet joint is a combination of a steroid and an anesthetic.

> **THE BACK AND BEYOND**
>
> Sometimes, injections are used for sacroiliac (SI) joint pain. The SI joint is the juncture of your sacrum and hip bones and it's often an underdiagnosed source of back pain. Savvy doctors, however, know to look to this area for diagnosis and treatment.

These injections require the use of radiological fluoroscopy, basically a fancy X-ray that allows physicians to see real-time images of your bones and the needle as it goes in. Sometimes dye is injected around the nerve to show that the medication is flowing in the right area.

Epidural Steroid Injections

For those suffering from sharp, shooting pain, such as from sciatica, this may be recommended. The injection tends to work best when received within the first few months of pain. Studies show if you wait much longer, it's less effective.

A steroid is injected into the epidural space outside the spinal canal. A specialist must be specifically trained to do this procedure. Injecting meds in this area affects a number of nerves. The sciatic nerve is composed of several nerves whose roots are in the lower back, which is why this injection can be particularly effective for sciatic pain.

As with facet-joint injection, this procedure is done under fluoroscopy. Patients might feel better right away because of the numbing effect of the anesthetic, but it usually takes several days to feel the full effect of an epidural steroid. Injections may last about six months, and patients generally require another dose or two before the natural healing process of the body has taken place. Other times, the injection may only last a few days.

> **WATCH YOUR BACK**
>
> Steroids used for back pain are not the same as anabolic steroids used to bulk up muscles. So although there's no risk of turning into the Incredible Hulk, there are side effects to steroids. Overuse can depress immune function, destroy joint cartilage, and cause bones to become brittle.

Nerve-Root Blocks

Epidural injections affect a broader range of nerves, whereas nerve-root blocks target specific nerves. Otherwise, the procedure is similar in use of technology and medication.

When injecting a nerve-root block, the specialist first inserts an anesthetic to see whether the appropriate nerve has been reached. He or she must place the needle carefully at the site where the nerve exits the spine. The nerve itself is not injected; rather, the needle enters the space around the nerve. If the anesthetic stops the pain, the right nerve has been found and steroid is then injected into the site. Sometimes selective nerve-root blocks are used to help diagnose which nerve is symptomatic and to help direct future treatments such as surgery for specific nerve-root decompression. It can take several attempts to find the right nerve, but the process isn't lengthy. It takes only about 10 minutes or so to test each injected nerve root.

Nerve-root blocks can be more effective because the exact nerve involved in the pain has been found and treated. Most of the time, this procedure is used to treat nerve pain and sciatica.

Electrical Stimulation Therapies

Isn't it shocking how many options there are in treating back pain? (Sorry, we couldn't resist.) The theory behind using electrical impulses isn't far-fetched when we consider that the body itself produces electrochemical impulses. Pain is a traveler on the electro-chemical highway. Blocking pain signals with electrical impulses seems to work for some people. The research on the subject is mixed, however.

But don't worry, you won't shock yourself silly with these options. In fact, the downside with external stimulation is that it may not work.

Transcutaneous Electrical Nerve Stimulation

Transcutaneous electrical nerve stimulation (TENS) has been around for more than 30 years. Electrical impulses are sent through the skin via small pads attached to the body. The pads are linked by wires to a portable device (battery-operated and plugged-in versions are available). Physical therapists or other rehab specialists often use TENS. They place the electrodes near the site of pain, and can control intensity of the electrical impulses. TENS allegedly works by stimulating nerve fibers that turn off pain signals (à la the gate control theory discussed in Chapter 2). TENS may trigger the release of endorphins, a natural painkiller producer by the body. You can even purchase a TENS device for home use.

Percutaneous Electrical Nerve Stimulation

Percutaneous means under the skin. This device uses needles instead of pads to deliver electrical impulses. Some say this works better because the electrical charges can more easily reach nerves.

Bracing

As the name implies, a brace helps support your body. These help support and correct your posture. For example, a brace that helps keep your shoulders back and your upper spine erect can be helpful when you spend long hours at the computer. Braces also restrict movement, which can be helpful if you're recovering from surgery and you need stability to heal. Braces can also constrain muscles in your back if you are lifting. That way, the muscles constrict in a fixed plane and do not bulge out, causing abnormal strain.

In general, though, most doctors recommend bracing for only short periods of time. The goal is to train your muscles to support your spine as nature intended.

The Least You Need to Know

- Physical therapy helps you recover and learn how to move properly, thereby keeping your back healthier for life.

- Minimizing pain can require different kinds of medications. Prescription medications can be for pain, inflammation, or both.

- Injecting medicine directly into the site of pain can be effective when oral medications aren't doing the job.

- Devices that emit electrical impulses can reduce pain for some people.

- It's important to build muscles to support the spine, but sometimes braces can lend extra support during the rehabilitation phase, especially after surgery.

Complementary and Alternative Options

In This Chapter

- Key terms related to complementary and alternative options
- The many options that have scientific evidence, as well as those that have a long history that predates conventional medicine
- Commonly recommended alternative and complementary treatments for back care

The National Institutes of Health define complementary and alternative medicine (CAM) as a group of diverse health-care systems, practices, and products that are not generally considered part of conventional medicine. These include everything from acupuncture to ultrasound. Some of these treatments have medically recognized scientific research to back up claims; many do not. But even though research may be lacking, practices such as acupuncture have been around for thousands of years. They are quite valid to the many people who find relief from them.

Conventional medicine has begun to accept and even recommend some CAM practices, enough that a new branch of medicine has recently been established called integrative medicine. This discipline combines conventional and CAM treatments for which there is evidence of safety and effectiveness. Practitioners are medical doctors with education in CAM treatments. Among the most well-known integrative medicine doctors is best-selling author Dr. Andrew Weil.

His many publications and popular website have done much to encourage the public and other medical professionals to look beyond conventional medicine as the only healing modality. (Modality refers to any therapeutic technique or agent. A massage therapist may use several modalities, such as Swedish and deep tissue massage; a conventional doctor may prescribe pain and anti-inflammatory medicines to treat back pain.)

In this chapter, we cover the most commonly accepted CAM treatments for back care and treatment. You don't need a doctor's prescription or permission to try these options. However, we highly recommend that you tell your doctor about any and all treatments you do try. Likewise, you should tell your CAM practitioner about any conventional treatments, especially medicines that you are taking.

Multiple Medicines

Let's take a moment and define these different schools of medicine. Alternative medicine includes therapies and practices considered outside of conventional medicine such as massage and acupuncture. In general, alternative medicine is less invasive (meaning not penetrating the body, such as with surgery), gentler, and based on nature (such as herbal medicine). The practice tends toward holistic practices in that it evaluates the whole person: mind, body, and spirit. Alternative medicines are sometimes used in place of conventional medicine—for example, taking ginger to calm nausea instead of Pepto Bismol.

Complementary medicine refers to using alternative medicine in combination with conventional practices. These may be patient-selected or doctor-recommended—for example, using massage and chiropractic along with ibuprofen to treat back pain.

Conventional medicine refers to the system with which you're most familiar, in which medical doctors and other health-care professionals (nurses, pharmacists, and therapists) diagnose and treat symptoms and diseases using drugs, radiation, or surgery. It's also called allopathic medicine, mainstream medicine, and Western medicine.

Integrative medicine is a branch of conventional medicine that integrates CAM techniques for whose effectiveness there has been ample scientific evidence. It's a fast-growing field. You're likely to see many major medical hospitals featuring integrative medicine centers. Take note, however, that even though an integrative medical doctor recommends a treatment, patients often pay out of pocket for many services. Fortunately, that's starting to change as some insurance policies are covering services such as therapeutic massage, chiropractic treatments, and biofeedback.

Chiropractic

Some people refer to chiropractic treatments as getting their "backs cracked." And indeed, if you get a treatment (called an adjustment or manipulation), you may hear a popping sound similar to cracking your knuckles. But don't worry; nothing is breaking. Although it's not absolutely known what causes the sound, the prevailing theory is that it is trapped air being released from joints. It's not painful, but it can be a little disconcerting to hear.

The idea behind chiropractic treatments is to realign your spine. Vertebral bones can slightly shift out of place for a number of reasons, including poor posture, repetitive physical stress, or injury. Chiropractors manually readjust the spine to move the bones back where they belong.

WATCH YOUR BACK

Although chiropractic treatments are generally considered safe, they are not for everyone. You should avoid chiropractic treatment if you have any disease that weakens bones, such as osteoporosis, rheumatoid arthritis, or bone cancer.

Your first visit to a chiropractor is likely to be lengthy. It should be. Similar to conventional doctors, chiropractors will chart the location and sensation of your pain. He or she should take a complete health record and administer a thorough physical exam. Chiropractors will want to look at your posture as you walk, sit, stand, and lie down.

After the chiropractor diagnoses your situation, he or she will adjust your spine. An adjustment is typically done on what's called a drop table. It looks like a massage table with a small, built-in platform that moves up and down a few inches. You'll be asked to lie face up or down or on your side. The chiropractor uses his or her hands and the sudden force of the drop table to move your spine back into place. The chiropractor will also use his or her arm strength to twist and turn your spine in various directions. It is a very physical experience!

Many people report immediate relief after a treatment, although it can take several treatments to get back into alignment. Beware of chiropractors who want to sell you a package of ongoing treatments on your first visit. See how you feel afterward before committing to a series.

There is some debate over how effective chiropractic care is in the long term. Some people question whether simple manipulation and realignment can fix what's wrong when there is nothing done to prevent recurrence. Muscles move bones. If you don't address the underlying issue of why your bones shifted, you're not doing enough to prevent recurrence. That's why a wise chiropractor will include exercises and postural awareness as part of an overall program to maintain spine health.

Acupuncture/Acupressure

These treatments are a branch of traditional Chinese medicine. In the United States, they are generally practiced as stand-alone treatments by a person trained in acupuncture/acupressure. Most states regulate acupuncture as a licensed specialty.

THE BACK AND BEYOND

Some research has shown that acupuncture works by stimulating the release of the body's natural pain-killing chemicals.

The philosophy behind acupuncture/acupressure is the same, based on the idea of energy that flows through all life. This life energy is called *chi* or *qi* (pronounced *chee*). Life energy is believed to have oppositional forces called *yin* and *yang*. In simple terms, yin is associated with passive, absorbing, and yielding qualities and yang as having more assertive and penetrating attributes. One is not better than the other; they are complementary. When these forces are out of balance, a health problem develops. Acupuncture/acupressure helps release blockages to restore natural flow.

Life energy flows through the body along what are called meridian lines. There are 14 main lines and hundreds more. Acupuncture/ acupressure practitioners determine where the energy is blocked along the meridians and they seek to release it. Acupressure does this by applying pressure (generally with a thumb); acupuncture does so with needles. The needles are hair-thin and do not hurt when inserted. The needles usually stay in place for about 20 minutes. In the case of acupressure, the practitioner holds a point for a length of time, then releases it. In either case, the person receiving the treatment usually feels quite relaxed. Several sessions are generally recommended.

Acupuncture has been practiced in Asia for more than 4,000 years. It's made its way into the United States during the past few decades. Its popularity is rising, especially as more conventional doctors recommend it for everything from back pain to headaches to carpal tunnel. We recommend trying it!

Massage

There's nothing like a good massage to relax you. And a fair bit of science shows that massage does more than just help you relax, it can help relieve chronic and acute back pain by releasing natural pain-reducing chemicals. Massage has its roots in Chinese medicine. Like acupuncture/acupressure, it's been practiced as a healing art for thousands of years. In the late nineteenth century, it was popularized in the Western world by a Swede named Per Henrik Ling.

There are different types of massage, or modalities. Most are based on what's called Swedish massage, which has four main techniques: stroking, tapping, kneading, and friction (basically small circular movements). Pressure varies according to a client's needs. It is extremely important that you communicate with your massage therapist during your session. Good therapists can sense when the pressure may be too much, as they'll feel your muscles tense instead of release. But they are not mind readers. If it hurts, tell them. Conversely, it you want more pressure, say so.

Massage is typically done while you are nude, although some people prefer to leave on underclothes. The therapist leaves the room while you disrobe and reenters when you are on the massage table covered with a sheet. The therapist uncovers only the portions of the body being massaged. Scented or nonscented oil is applied to your skin to help the therapist massage your body. If you have allergies, ask the therapist about the products he or she is using.

The massage room should be warm and dimly lit with perhaps some relaxing music. Again, communicate if you prefer silence or if the room temperature is not to your liking. Relaxation is very important in releasing tense muscles and you can't do it if you're annoyed by some environmental aspect.

THE BACK AND BEYOND

Shiatsu is a modality that combines acupressure with massage. You wear loose clothing and lie on a soft mat on the floor. The practitioner works on your body's meridian points using his or her fingers, knuckles, elbows, and sometimes feet. He or she will likely do a thorough inter-view asking you about your lifestyle and specifics about your back pain.

Good massage therapists will do a thorough health interview (also known as an intake) and keep your chart on file. They will also prep you with tips on making the most of your massage before, during, and after your session. It will likely require several sessions to find maximum benefit, but what an enjoyable way to bring relief to your body! Therapeutic massage is frequently covered by many insurance policies, but you'll need a referral from your doctor. Also, you may be restricted to particular massage therapists. As always, find out about the particulars of policy benefits before assuming coverage.

Biofeedback

You may have heard stories about ancient yogis who were able to reduce their blood pressure and heart rate through meditation. It's true. They can do it and so can you. We can all control some physiological responses. With biofeedback, you can see it happen before your very eyes—and you don't have to be a yogi meditating in a cave for eight hours a day.

A biofeedback machine measures physiological states such as body temperature, blood pressure, and electrical activity of muscles. Small pads with electrodes are placed on your body and then plugged into a machine. A monitor reports the results instantly through blinking lights and/or beeping sounds. When electrodes are placed on back muscles that are tense, the lights blink at a faster rate. As you practice relaxation techniques, the blinks and beeps slow down, showing you how your thoughts have changed your physiological responses. Pretty neat, huh?

> **BODY WISE**
>
> With back pain, especially chronic conditions, it's important to address underlying structural problems (such as facet-joint disease and disc degeneration). CAM treatments should be a part of an overall approach to back care rather than a stand-alone approach.

Typically, you'll see a biofeedback therapist (who could be a nurse or physical therapist) who will help you with the machine and coach you through relaxation techniques. The ultimate goal is to wean you off the machine and simply do these techniques when you feel stressed out or when back pain increases. It will require several sessions to really learn how to exert this kind of control. You are essentially learning a new behavior, and changing behavior takes time. The instant feedback of the machine, however, can speed along the change process, especially for people who "have to see it to believe it." Also know that you can purchase home versions of biofeedback machines.

Ultrasound

In this therapy, an ultrasound machine applies high-frequency sound waves to tense muscles in an effort to release them. The treatment is painless and you can't hear the sound waves (although you'll feel a tingling sensation). A person trained in the use of ultrasound therapy (usually a physical therapist) will administer the treatment.

Like oil helps massage therapists glide their hands over your skin, ultrasound therapy uses a cool gel for the same purpose. The ultrasound therapist applies this gel, then treats an area by moving a wandlike device in a circular motion on your back. The sound waves are absorbed deep into your tissues. They also heat those tissues, which promotes circulation. Sometimes, a topical anti-inflammatory is mixed with the gel so the medication can be absorbed more deeply.

Ultrasound waves can cause heating in a similar manner to microwave ovens, albeit milder. This heat improves circulation. Some experts believe that ultrasound does little more than, say, a heating pad, and is a comparatively expensive treatment.

Inversion Therapy

Turning the body upside down to promote a healing effect is nothing new. It's why yogis do headstands, handstands, and other upside-down postures. From the standpoint of pure physics, inversions counteract the effects of gravity. All day long, gravity is pressing down on your body, including the spine and intervertebral discs. When we turn upside down, the spine is decompressed and surrounding muscles are lengthened. You don't have to stand on your head (and you shouldn't, frankly, as it applies way too much pressure for your neck). And proponents say you don't have to be completely upside down to experience the benefits. Simply having your torso below your waist will give you the effects, even at –5 or –10 degrees. We suggest this gentler approach of inclining a few degrees back rather than hanging completely upside down. For those with back problems, hanging fully upside down can overly stress discs and facet joints and create too much slack within joints.

You could hang upside down in any number of ways, but it's most common (and easiest) to do so with an inversion table. These tables allow you to control how far over you will go. You lie down, securely fasten your legs, and tilt the machine backward. You can move upside down in small increments from as little as a few degrees to fully upside down.

THE BACK AND BEYOND

The intervertebral disc is the largest organ in the body *without blood supply*. Most lumbar discs are the size of a watch face and have no arteries going to them. Discs rely on the surrounding bone for nutrients. These nutrients percolate into the disc much like coffee going through a filter. Some studies suggest that pulling the bones apart through inversion therapy may help this process by drawing more fluid into the disc. This allows greater nutrient flow and improves disc hydration and height.

Inversion tables are primarily devices that you purchase for home use. Some physical therapists or exercise professionals may also have them. Try before you buy. And talk to your doctor before doing inversion therapy. You shouldn't invert your body if you have certain medical conditions such as high blood pressure, detached retina, or glaucoma. Inversion therapy can also exacerbate laxity of the joints, or spondylolisthesis.

Prolotherapy

This treatment is considered an alternative but isn't in the same category of the other treatments we've discussed in this chapter. It's not a holistic treatment. It's an invasive medical procedure.

The goal of prolotherapy is to stimulate the growth of tendons and ligaments. As you might recall from Chapter 3, tendons attach muscles to bone, and ligaments attach bone to bone. These tissues help stabilize your spine. Prolotherapy is most commonly tried for those who have degenerative disc disease, a condition that causes the discs to shrink. When intervertebral discs lose their height, ligaments and tendons can slacken, no longer providing needed support to the spine.

Prolotherapy is based on injecting mild solutions (typically sugar water) into affected tendons and ligaments. This is an example of how the inflammatory response is indeed the body's way of healing itself. The injected solution causes localized inflammation at the site of the weakened tendons or ligaments. Increased blood supply floods the area along with nutrients to stimulate the tissue to repair itself. The new growth provides better support for the spine. It may take a number of injections for this therapy to work.

Although some patients report relief, most physicians are skeptical. The argument they make is that most injured tissue is already irritated, and irritating it more won't encourage the body to respond. Chronic pain patients will try anything, and although some find relief, the actual effectiveness of prolotherapy remains inconclusive.

The Least You Need to Know

- Alternative treatments for back care come in many varieties; some have more scientific research behind them than others.
- Some alternative treatments are ancient healing practices that have provided relief to people for centuries.
- Most, but not all, complementary and alternative medicine (CAM) practices take a holistic (mind, body, and spirit) approach to healing.
- Many conventional medical doctors recommend some CAM practices for back pain.
- Alternative treatments can be doctor-recommended or you can try them on your own.

Chronic Pain Management

In This Chapter

- Treatments for chronic pain management are many and multidisciplinary
- Scientific researchers learn more about how chronic pain manifests in bodies and minds
- Dealing with emotions can help you better manage your pain

Chronic pain is typically defined as pain that persists for longer than six months. What makes it especially frustrating is that we don't really know why this pain persists even after an injury has healed. It's speculated that for some reason, the body's nervous system continues to send pain signals even when the root cause has been identified and addressed.

Successful chronic pain management is a multidimensional approach that includes medication and physical and psychological treatments. Patients with chronic pain typically see doctors who specialize in chronic pain management. Pain management specialists include experts from a variety of disciplines who come at pain from different directions. They include specially trained psychiatrists, neurologists, anesthesiologists, and physiatrists (medical rehab specialists).

Pain and Your Brain

As we discussed in Chapter 2, sudden and intense acute pain can cause the nervous system to become overly sensitive, turning the slightest discomfort into extreme pain. New discoveries in how the brain processes memory and learning, called *neuroplasticity*, are shedding light on how the nervous system and brain work together. As researchers understand more about neuroplasticity and how it may relate to chronic pain, they can develop better ways of stopping chronic pain before it starts. Until then, there are treatments and techniques that can help you deal with ongoing pain.

Neuroplasticity is a relatively new concept explaining how our nervous system participates in memory. When we learn new concepts or experience events, nerves send signals to one another, creating connections. Through repetition and intensity, lasting connections among neural pathways are made. For example, such pathways were created when you learned to walk, which makes walking second nature. The nervous system remembers all kinds of things, including pain. When the pain is especially intense and/or long lasting, the central nervous system (brain and spinal cord) can be reprogrammed. It's possible that the neurons that prevent pain signals actually die. There are no longer the natural checks and balances for pain signals, allowing pain-producing signals to flow freely. This results in chronic pain.

Medications

Unfortunately for many chronic pain sufferers, over-the-counter medications generally don't do enough. Such patients typically need prescription medication. Doctors will start with lower doses of prescriptions, an especially important step because chronic pain patients will need to take these drugs continuously.

Keep in mind that pain meds don't cure; they temper pain and help people lead more normal lives. The medications for chronic pain are similar to those taken for acute or postsurgical circumstances. Because different meds do different things, they may be prescribed in combination. Chronic pain meds include antidepressants, neuropathic agents, muscle relaxants, nonsteroidal anti-inflammatory drugs (NSAIDs), steroids, and opiates:

- Antidepressants can block pain signals from reaching the brain. These drugs may also help your body release endorphins, your own natural pain-fighting chemicals. Of course, chronic pain may also lead to depression, which is another reason your doctor might prescribe this type of medication.

- Neuropathic agents address chronic pain problems that stem from nerve damage or hypersensitive nerves. These drugs change the way pain signals travel and how they are interpreted in the brain.

- Muscle relaxants are prescribed when the pain is from muscle sprains and strains.

- Nonsteroidal anti-inflammatory drugs (NSAIDs), as the name implies, reduce inflammation. When tissue swelling and pain-signaling molecules diminish, pain is reduced as well.

- Steroids also reduce inflammation, but they are much more powerful drugs with greater side effects. Doctors typically prescribe these only after NSAIDs have failed.

- Opiates work by blocking pain signals from reaching the brain. The problem with opiates is not so much addiction as it is habituation, or tolerance. This means the body metabolizes or uses up the medication quicker and you need an increasingly higher dose the longer you are on it.

BODY WISE

Conventional medical researchers state that the ancient Chinese medical treatment of acupuncture can significantly reduce pain. The findings were published in the May 11, 2009, issue of the *Archives of Internal Medicine*. More than 600 patients with chronic lower back pain were included in what was the largest study of its kind in the United States. The study found that acupuncture was effective for treating back pain, but the researchers couldn't explain exactly why it worked.

Chronic Pain Management Continuum

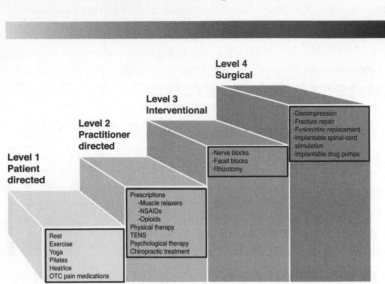

Chronic pain management continuum.

Spinal-Cord Stimulation

This therapy involves using low-voltage electricity to block the transmission of pain through the spinal cord before it reaches the brain. A small pulse generator connects to spaghetti-like electrodes implanted under the skin along the surface of the spinal cord. Here the electricity overrides the normal pain transmission and replaces it with a gentle, prickly sensation. On the physiological level, it is much like the effect of rubbing your foot after you stub your toe. By rubbing, you are mechanically stimulating nerves that block pain. The spinal-cord stimulator does so electronically.

Still, spinal-cord stimulation devices are not for everyone. Doctors recommend them only after other therapies have failed. You cannot get magnetic resonance imaging (MRI) scans with them in and sometimes scar tissue blocks their effectiveness. They are also quite costly, priced at about $20,000.

If it is the chosen route, patients are thoroughly screened to ensure that the device is appropriate for their lifestyle. A trial device is first implanted to confirm the therapy will work. If it does, the surgeon implants a permanent device.

Intrathecal Pumps

Unlike oral pain medication that has to go through the digestive system, the pump (an implanted device) delivers medication directly to the spinal canal. Site-specific delivery results in fewer side effects than are common from powerful pain meds such as morphine. The amount and frequency of the medication are determined by a computer chip. As with spinal-cord stimulators, neurosurgeons first test this approach with a temporary device.

The downfall of this approach is that all the medication is stored within the implanted device. Typically, medication is refilled every few months. It's rare, but a malfunction could cause the pump to stop or overdeliver medication. If complications do occur, the surgeon can completely reverse the treatment by removing the pump. The problem of tolerance to the medication and some of the sedating side effects can still occur. On the positive side, the majority of patients report immediate relief.

Emotional and Spiritual Therapy

Chronic pain interrupts life as you know it. It affects body, mind, and spirit. A study reported in a 2008 edition of the *Journal of Neuroscience* said that chronic pain impacts overall brain function. That includes your emotions. The researchers compared people with chronic back pain to those without pain.

Through the use of MRIs, researchers could see that those with chronic pain had continuous activity in the part of the brain that's associated with emotions. This overactivity leads chronic pain sufferers to experience more stress, depression, anxiety, and sleeplessness. If your brain is so busy processing chronic pain, your mind is not freed up to get adequate rest.

That's why getting the emotional and spiritual help you need is as important as any pain medication. Depression and anxiety often accompany chronic pain, so talking to a psychologist trained in pain management is a good choice. Alternately or additionally, seeking the counsel of a trusted religious or spiritual leader is also wise. There is no one correct method to deal with the emotional distress that chronic pain can create. The best method is the one that most resonates with you.

A psychologist trained in pain management will listen and understand your pain in a way that family and friends perhaps may not. His or her office is a place where you can freely express what you're feeling, knowing that you won't be negatively judged. Sometimes it's a huge relief simply to be heard. And by listening to your challenges and your feelings, a psychologist can devise a plan for your specific needs.

Stress, of course, is a huge part of chronic pain. Through psychologists and others, you can learn to reduce stress. Spiritual counselors can help you find peace through prayer. Other mind/body experts such as those specializing in Eastern disciplines (such as yoga or tai chi) can help you find release through meditative techniques.

BODY WISE

Massage, exercise, and physical therapy are helpful for chronic pain management. Massage can help reduce stress and release pain-relieving endorphins. Exercise can also release endorphins and help you build muscles to support your spine. Physical therapy helps you create and maintain the right posture and develops an exercise program tailored for your specific needs.

Emotions cannot be disregarded. As much as we might like to simply pop a pill to numb symptoms, it's a short-term solution that ultimately will not be enough to manage long-term pain. Fortunately, the subject of emotions is no longer taboo in our society. Emotions shape and govern our experiences, our health, and our quality of life. That's why learning to work with emotions is an especially crucial piece in the chronic pain management puzzle.

The Least You Need to Know

- Reasons for chronic pain are unclear, but there are many treatments to help people lead a better quality of life.
- Our nervous system has a pain memory. When overstimulated, it can lead to chronic pain.
- Successfully treating chronic pain requires a multifaceted approach that includes the body, mind, and spirit.

The Last Resort: Surgery

In This Chapter

- Back conditions and the surgical options that can help heal them
- New advances that have made back surgeries less invasive
- Post-op care, including motions to avoid and physical activity to do

Back surgery is usually an elective surgery. The exception is when there is an emergency or rare condition such as a tumor, infection, cauda equina syndrome, or trauma that causes damage to the spinal cord. But these situations are truly rare. Generally, it is up to you and your doctor to determine whether or not back surgery is the right choice for your particular condition.

Most back surgery is done to relieve pressure from the nerve or stabilize a segment of the spine. Diagnostic tests will confirm whether a particular root is at fault. The causes of pinched nerves are many, including vertebral fractures, bulging discs, or bone spurs, just to name a few. Different reasons, different surgical options.

To follow are among the most commonly performed back surgeries. Surgeons who perform them are either neurosurgeons (specializing in the nervous system) or orthopedic surgeons (those who specialize in bones), ideally ones who focus on the spine instead of general orthopedics.

Back Surgery Is No Guarantee

Statistics show that many back surgeries successfully reduce or eliminate pain as intended. However, failure rates can be anywhere from 10 to 40 percent. In medical parlance, it's called *failed back-surgery syndrome (FBSS)*. In those cases, patients may undergo yet another procedure or try a different approach. Back surgeries can fail for many reasons. Problems can include scar tissue, instability issues caused by some decompressions, or unrealistic expectations of what the surgery could fix. The biggest contributor to FBSS is persistent pain.

> **DEFINITIONS**
>
> **Failed back-surgery syndrome (FBSS)** is the term used when patients continue to experience pain after the surgery. According to research from the National Institutes of Health, the incidence of failed back-surgery syndrome is about 40 percent.

With an elective procedure, you have time to research. Consider your options, realistically understand the potential outcomes, and evaluate surgeons very carefully. A qualified surgeon should be doing at least 100 cases per year. He or she should also be able to answer all your questions candidly and thoroughly and shed light on what to expect after surgery.

Also know that good surgeons are not intimidated when you want to get a second opinion. In fact, many recommend it. Of course, all surgeries carry some risk. Ask about both the risks and benefits. And be wary of anyone who promises to relieve all of your pain.

Decompressive

As you might recall from Chapter 3, 31 pairs of nerve roots exit from the spinal cord through spaces between the vertebrae. When those spaces are compromised, nerves can be compressed, which equals pain. Conditions that can compress nerves include:

- Spinal stenosis: A narrowing of the spinal canal

- Degenerative disc disease: Loss of fluid in the intervertebral discs

- Herniated disc: The bulging or rupturing of an intervertebral disc

- Bone spurs: Extra growth on vertebra often due to osteoarthritis

- Spondylosis: Spinal osteoarthritis causing joint dysfunction

THE BACK AND BEYOND

As spinal root nerves branch out, they become like a fine web of nerves distributed throughout the body. That's why you might feel what is called referred pain (pain felt in one part of the body when the source of irritation is actually located elsewhere). For example, if a nerve root exiting the lower back is pinched, you might feel pain or tingling down your leg. Sometimes it might be numbness or weakness, not pain. Releasing the compressed nerve usually gets rid of pain and normal sensation returns.

Discectomy

This procedure removes the part of your intervertebral disc that is pressing on a nerve. There are three general types: classic discectomy, microdiscectomy, and percutaneous discectomy. The main variable among them is the size of the incision. The choice depends on your unique situation. Although percutaneous discectomy is the least invasive, it is also the least effective for large herniations.

Surgical imaging technology has enabled surgeons to perform more advanced, less invasive procedures (with smaller incisions). Surgeons can now use microscopes, magnifying *loupes*, or endoscopes to see the spine in greater detail.

DEFINITIONS

Surgeons commonly use surgical **loupes,** which are magnifying lenses worn like glasses. These are often custom made to take into account the surgeon's vision.

Percutaneous discectomy is the least invasive and often done as an outpatient procedure. The surgeon makes a small puncture through the skin and, using X-ray technology and a needle, suctions out troublesome disc material. These surgeries are usually done when disc herniations have not ruptured but only bulged. Only select patients are ideal candidates for this procedure and the long-term effectiveness of it has been called into question.

In microdiscectomy, the surgeon makes a small incision (about an inch or two long). Either tubular or blade-based retractors are placed through the incision to push aside muscle and soft tissue. A small section of bone and ligament is removed to expose the disc. Then a magnifying device (surgical loupes or a microscope) is used to see the damaged disc more easily. Disc fragments are removed from around the nerve. Some additional removal of fragments within the disc space is done to reduce recurrence of herniation.

A classic discectomy requires a larger incision, but provides better visualization of the tissue. In most cases, however, a microdiscectomy can provide the surgeon with enough visualization to do the job adequately. Also, understand that in a discectomy the entire disc is usually not removed. The annulus (outer portion) and a part of the nucleus (inner portion) are left intact to support surrounding vertebrae.

Foraminotomy

There is a space between every pair of vertebrae called the intervertebral *foramina* or neural foramina. When disc, ligament, or bone spurs creep into the space, the nerves within can get squeezed. This procedure involves removing part of the vertebral bone or excess tissue (such as the disc or ligaments) to create a larger space for the nerve root.

DEFINITIONS

In anatomical terms, a **foramin** (the plural form of which is **foramina**) refers to any opening. It's usually in reference to a space within or between bones, but it can mean a natural opening within tissues as well.

To reach the intervertebral foramina, an incision is made in the back and muscles are separated and retracted much like in the microdiscectomy procedure described in the preceding section. Excess tissue and/or bone are cut away until the desired opening has been created and the nerve is no longer compressed.

Laminotomy and Laminectomy

The spinal canal may narrow due to spinal stenosis, spondylolisthesis, or bone spurs. This procedure widens the space of the spinal canal by removing a section of bone called the lamina. A laminotomy creates an opening in the lamina; laminectomy is the removal of the lamina and/or a portion of it. Depending on how much of the spinal canal has been compromised, one vertebra or several may need to be trimmed. If a significant amount of bone has been removed, the area may be too unstable. The spine may require stabilization by spinal fusion (see the next section).

As scary as it may sound to have the top of your vertebral bones cut off, know that the spinal cord won't be as exposed as you might imagine. The spinal cord is surrounded by bones on either side and it's also encased by muscles and connective tissue. Patients with a laminectomy can typically resume normal activity with no restrictions after a period of healing.

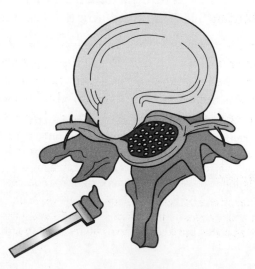

Laminectomy.

Stabilizing

Any number of conditions may destabilize the spine: arthritis, removal of intervertebral disc, or osteoporosis. Regardless, if the spine becomes too unstable, conditions and pain may worsen. The goal of this type of surgery is to stabilize the vertebrae.

> **BODY WISE**
>
> If you are contemplating surgery, there's no better time to get in good physical condition. The stronger your back and abdominal muscles are presurgery, the easier rehab will be.

Fusion

You might hold the common misconception that fusions are undesirable and limit mobility. And it's true that fusion will limit some mobility when you compare it to someone who has no spine problems. But this procedure can be a saving grace, especially when your joints have totally deteriorated and bone spurs obstruct nerve passages.

Fusion is actually what the body does naturally in response to some traumatic conditions. Surgery moves the process along more quickly and also benefits patients by releasing trapped nerves. Some people may find their mobility is actually better after fusion because they are no longer in pain. The painful segment that kept them from moving at all is now immobile, leaving the rest of the spine free to bend and twist.

> **WATCH YOUR BACK**
>
> Traditional fusion can create excess pressure on surrounding vertebrae, which can lead to disc problems elsewhere in the spine. This is called adjacent segment disease. It is one reason surgeons are reluctant to do multilevel fusions. The longer a fused segment, the more pressure on neighboring levels, and with time there may be a need for further surgery.

In fusion, the goal is to immobilize the painful segment and bridge the two vertebrae with bone. First, surgeons stabilize the spine with titanium or stainless steel rods and screws. This acts as an internal brace. Bone graft is then inserted to grow between the two vertebrae. Bone graft material is obtained from the bony decompression, the patient's own hip (although this is rarely done these days), a donor, or a genetically engineered source. It takes about six months for the spinal bones to fuse together.

Dynamic Stabilization

Sometimes decompression may make the spine unstable but a fusion is not needed. Dynamic stabilization reinforces the spine to allow more natural motion than a fusion. This is still an investigational procedure but it may reduce the risk of adjacent segment disease.

One benefit of dynamic stabilization is that it provides support without fusion, so ideally little motion is lost. The goal is to lessen the chance of the next vertebral segment from the spine wearing out as quickly because you can distribute forces. The downsides are that this procedure is not recognized as a standard of care, so most insurance companies do not cover it.

Only a few surgeons in the United States perform dynamic stabilization. There is some concern that the hardware may loosen over time because there is motion there. Once a fusion has healed, there is no motion, so hardware does not loosen. Also, dynamic stabilization allows motion at the treated level, which may cause pain. In some cases, a fusion eliminates the painful motion and may be a better option.

Disc Replacement

When a disc has to be entirely removed, something has to replace it or else the vertebrae will sit on top of one another. In cases of severe disc degeneration, the disc is practically gone anyway. Any movement of the spine will cause bone-on-bone friction. So the patient's choice is either fusion or disc replacement.

Developing an artificial disc has been in the works for decades. Creating a device that works for a diverse population and can replicate the natural movements allowed by real discs is challenging, to say the least, but progress has been made. In 2004, the CHARITÈ Artificial Disc became the first artificial disc to be approved by the U.S. Food and Drug Administration as a surgical treatment for patients suffering with single-level degenerative disc disease in the lower back.

Unfortunately, artificial discs, particularly in the lumbar spine, perform no better than fusion in long-term studies. In fact, they have been associated with more complications, because they allow movement and are subject to mechanical failure. Because of this, few insurance companies in the United States cover this procedure.

Although not right for everyone or every condition, artificial discs do help mimic the movement of a real intervertebral disc. Two metal plates with a plastic core replace the natural disc and enable the spine to move.

Fracture Repair

Vertebra can fracture from trauma or tumor. For patients with weak bones from osteoporosis or from steroids, the trauma causing the fracture can be as minor as coughing or reaching up to get a can of soup. Because these fractures are painful and the structural integrity of the bone is at risk, surgery is often considered. Vertebroplasty and kyphoplasty are two procedures that can help heal such fractures.

Vertebroplasty

Vertebroplasty is a minimally invasive outpatient procedure; just a small nick is made. A needle carrying injectable cement is guided by X-ray and inserted into the fractured vertebra. The cement fills in the microfractures within the vertebral body and stabilizes the bone. It takes about 10 minutes for the cement to set.

Kyphoplasty

This newer procedure is similar to vertebroplasty, but with a valuable advancement: restoring some bone height. Keep in mind that fractured vertebrae often collapse. This can create a domino effect and cause other vertebrae to misalign. With kyphoplasty, a temporary balloon is blown up inside the vertebrae to create space and restore some height. The balloon is removed, the open space is filled with cement, and the natural size of the vertebra is restored.

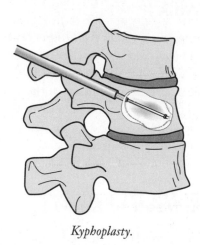

Kyphoplasty.

Post-Op Care

Recovering from surgery can take anywhere from a few weeks to several months. It depends on your procedure and your physical condition prior to your surgery. Post-op care will include physical therapy and your commitment to a continuing fitness program. Your doctor and post-op therapist will know what's best for your back after surgery. Don't ignore their advice, even if it feels like you're ready to run that marathon, or if you think you need more rest and they're urging you to get out of bed. Trust your doc and your physical therapist to get you safely back on track as quickly as possible.

Avoid the BLTs

You should avoid bending, lifting, and twisting in the early days following your surgery. It's not that you'll never do these motions again; it's just that they can put too much stress on healing tissues. Also, you may need to relearn how to do these motions in a way that causes less stress. Your physical therapist will help you learn proper body mechanics.

Walk, Walk, Walk

Now here's something you *can* do! Walking is great exercise. It's one of the easiest, most convenient ways to get activity into your day. The National Institutes for Health recommend that we get at least 30 minutes of physical activity most days of the week. And studies have shown that you get just as much benefit from several 10-minute bursts of activity as you do from one longer workout. Take a quick walk before work, at lunch, and after work, and you're done!

The Least You Need to Know

- Unless there is a medical emergency, back surgery is an elective procedure.
- Back surgery is generally done to release trapped nerves that cause pain.
- A variety of back surgeries are performed, but each basically does one of the following: decompresses, stabilizes, and repairs fractures. Some people need more than one type of procedure.
- Post-op care and therapy are crucial for proper healing and continued back health.

Hope on the Horizon

Chapter

10

In This Chapter

- Staying up to date on the latest and greatest treatments in back pain
- Promising new developments in back treatments, including facet-joint replacement and stem cell research
- Deciding whether a clinical trial is right for you

Back pain plagues people worldwide. As such, the medical community around the globe looks for new ways to treat and minimize symptoms. Promising technologies are being tested both in the United States and abroad, some with very good results, others still in refinement. In this chapter, we take a look at some of the most exciting developments. We'll also talk about clinical trials and how you can get involved.

Prominent Research and Development

Continuing medical education and scientific meetings showcase the latest and greatest in spine research. Physicians, surgeons, and researchers flock to these events to share their knowledge and learn from one another. Their meetings aren't open to the general public, but their websites are accessible. You can find press releases that summarize breakthroughs as well as detailed academic papers from presenters.

The organizations that present cutting-edge spine research include:

- The North American Spine Society

- The American Association of Neurological Surgeons

- The Congress of Neurological Surgeons

- The American Academy of Orthopedic Surgeons

- The International Society for the Advancement of Spine Surgery

- The International Spine Intervention Society

- Medline Plus, a website service of the National Institutes of Health and the National Library of Medicine, references findings from many of these organizations. At its homepage, look for the website's latest news link.

As you might realize by now, many tissues are involved in the spine, including nerves, bone, cartilage, ligaments, tendons, muscles, synovial fluid, joint capsules, and discs. There's a lot going on! Each tissue has a unique job to do, and yet they all must also work together. When there is an imbalance in their complex interaction, the result is often back pain, and treatment of one isolated component may not adequately address your pain. This is one reason that artificial disc replacement in the lumbar spine has not proven to be the panacea it was hoped to be. Some patients who have had artificial disc replacement still had facet dysfunction, joint inflammation, and other soft tissue anomalies. Disc replacement doesn't address these tissues and potentially can make them worse.

BODY WISE

Patients who seek help earlier for herniated discs fare better than patients who delay their care, say several leading studies. One such study compared 927 patients who sought treatment within six months of pain and 265 patients who waited longer than six months. Patients who waited longer had worse outcomes after both operative and non-operative treatments.

Disc Nucleus Replacement (DNR) and Prosthetic Disc Nucleus (PDN)

The DNR/PDN procedure is under investigational use in Europe, and is far from being approved by the Food and Drug Adminstration (FDA) here. The surgery replaces the problematic nucleus with an artificial one (typically an elastic-type material). Many kinks still need to be worked out. It's been difficult to keep the artificial disc in place and yet have it retain the mobility of a natural disc. To insert the disc, surgeons must create a hole and plug it. Finding a material that seals the hole and is also flexible has presented another hurdle.

It's commonly agreed that keeping as much natural tissue as possible is the best choice if such tissue isn't diseased. That's why researchers have been striving to create a replacement for only the innermost portion of the intervertebral disc, called the nucleus pulposus, which does the highly sophisticated job of absorbing the shock of movement in your spine. This is also the portion that can degenerate (lose its fluid) or bulge out and impinge nerves, causing pain. Replacing just this portion would allow surgeons to preserve the outer disc (made mostly of ligament) that securely connects two vertebras together.

WATCH YOUR BACK

When both the inner and outer disc parts are dysfunctional, fixing only one may not solve the problem.

Nucleus replacement also has the advantage of being a minimally invasive procedure. Conventional disc replacement, also known as total disc replacement (TDR), involves replacing the entire disc, including the cartilage endplates. As we just mentioned, keeping healthy tissues intact is better than replacing the full set of parts. In the lumbar spine, TDR has had mixed success. It's fallen out of favor with many surgeons and most insurers. No surgery is foolproof, and going back to try to fix a failed TDR is a risky procedure.

> **THE BACK AND BEYOND**
>
> Studies are under way to see whether stem cells can help regenerate disc material. This is particularly helpful to the hundreds of thousands of patients worldwide who suffer from degenerative discs. The biggest hurdle in disc regeneration is that the degenerated disc is a hostile environment. There is no blood supply, the disc is full of inflammatory proteins, and the environment is not favorable to repair, let alone new growth. Cartilage stem cells, which grow more favorably in damaged tissues with no blood supply, seem to hold the most promise at this time.

Facet Replacement

Facet joints, like any joints in the body, can degenerate due to arthritis, repetitive stress, or trauma. Changes in facet-joint function can pinch nerves and cause pain. Seen as a substitute for fusion, facet-joint replacement could allow patients more mobility without causing more stress to neighboring vertebrae, which is a problem with fusion.

A device under evaluation by the FDA is the facet replacement system ACADIA. This joint reconstruction device matches the size and shape of the facet joint and is designed to provide patients with pain relief, normal motion, and stability. A clinical trial evaluating the use of this device for lumbar spinal stenosis was under way in 2010. Two other similar devices were on hold at the time of publication.

Stem Cells

A first attempt to use bone stem cells to repair malformed, damaged bone was under way at the National Institutes of Health in 2010. Working with mice, a team of researchers pinpointed the location of bone-generating stem cells in the spine, at the ends of shins, and in other bones. The team also has identified factors that control the stem cells' growth. According to Alan E. Guttmacher, M.D., acting director of the Eunice Kennedy Shriver National Institute of Child Health and Human Development (NICHD), this enables researchers to explore ways to harness these cells so that ultimately they might be used to repair damaged or malformed bone, including the spine.

In Dusseldorf, Germany, the XCell-Center released encouraging results from a follow-up study of 140 spinal-cord injury patients treated with bone marrow stem cells in 2010. More than half of the participants improved after the treatment. Most patients reported some return of sensation to their hands, feet, arms, or trunk. Muscle strength and endurance also improved. For this procedure, the bone marrow cells are collected from the patients and then injected into their spinal fluid. The center is the first clinic in Europe to specialize in *regenerative medicine* using bone marrow stem cell therapy. Again, although the results are promising, they have yet to be validated, as most patients improve somewhat on their own after injury without stem cell treatment. As a study, it will be difficult to compare these treatments against a placebo to demonstrate their efficacy.

DEFINITIONS

Regenerative medicine refers to the field of tissue regeneration using stem cells. The body's ability to regenerate tissues is no longer the lore of science fiction. Stem cells can grow into different types of cells—they can become a muscle cell, a red blood cell, or a brain cell. After all, you have to remember that each complex cell in the human body originated from one fertilized egg cell. Experiments have shown that these miraculous cells can also repair or regenerate damaged tissues and restore organ function.

Although stem cells hold great promise in treating chronic disease, the growth factors and genetic modifications required to grow these cells are complex. Harnessing and managing this growth is even more daunting. Don't forget that tumors grow from cells that have simply lost their ability to self-regulate. Uncontrolled cell growth is what cancer is! Experimental stem cell growth can have unintentional and undesirable consequences such as scarring or matting of nerve fibers.

Thirty-Two–Channel Spinal-Cord Stimulation

We've already mentioned spinal-cord stimulation as a treatment for chronic pain. Like most things electronic and computerized, these devices are becoming smaller, smarter, and more sophisticated.

At the time of this publication, stimulators were limited to 16 contacts, or electrodes. Research is under way to double the capacity of these, just as computers get more memory and have expanded capabilities.

Cortical and Deep-Brain Stimulation

Patients with Parkinson's Disease have already seen impressive gains from electrodes planted deep within the brain to improve their function. Studies are under way to implant similar devices to block the perception of pain at the brain and consciousness levels. Similarly, electrodes placed on the surface of the brain can also blunt pain perception more specifically than can be accomplished in the spinal cord.

Experimental Treatments Abroad

Many patients are drawn to seek spine care overseas in hopes of getting the latest and greatest treatment. Although that does offer the promise of the latest technology, it is important to remember that complications can occur, and local physicians are often reluctant to pick up where foreign physicians have left off. Many of the experimental treatments are just that—experimental—often with less rigid study designs and shorter follow-up than are used by more conservative regulatory agencies such as the FDA. Likewise, although the FDA moves slowly to approve new techniques, Medicare and most insurance companies follow even slower. Remember, most techniques that have shown overwhelming success are readily and rapidly adopted worldwide.

If you do move forward, do plenty of research. Talk with other patients who have had the procedure. And have a local doctor in the know who's willing to help you should you need additional care when you come home.

Are Clinical Trials Right for You?

To figure out whether a medicine or a treatment will work on a wide variety of people, researchers go through vigorous testing processes. After animal and other studies, researchers move on to clinical trials, which test how effective a treatment is on people. Each trial follows a very specific protocol and study plan that details what researchers will do. These trials are regulated in the United States by the FDA.

Patients should be aware that these studies and their regulation are designed to protect patients. If a treatment is found to show phenomenal results and great promise, a humanitarian clause ends the study early and opens the eligibility for all patients to receive the treatment.

Finding and Qualifying for Clinical Trials

A good place to look for clinical trials is at clinicaltrials.gov. You can search on topics such as diseases, conditions, or trial locations. At any given time, you're likely to find hundreds of studies on back pain. Research topics can include anything from examining meditation's effect on back pain to the effectiveness of a new pain drug.

THE BACK AND BEYOND

Even if you don't want to participate in a clinical trial, you can see what's in the works and discover the outcome of particular trials. Clinicaltrials. gov posts information about studies that are recruiting, those that have been completed, and those that have published results.

You'll have to qualify for a study. Eligibility requirements may include age, gender, disease state, and medications taken. Some studies look for healthy recruits; others look for people with specific diseases or conditions. Researchers report the progress and outcomes of the clinical trials to various government agencies, medical journals, and scientific meetings. Your participation in a trial is kept confidential. No names appear in reports.

If you find a trial of interest, your next step is to contact the study's research staff and ask questions about specific trials. The National Institutes of Health recommend you ask questions such as the following:

- Why do researchers believe the experimental treatment being tested may be effective? Has it been tested before?

- What kinds of tests and experimental treatments are involved?

- How do the possible risks, side effects, and benefits in the study compare with my current treatment?

- How might this trial affect my daily life?

- Who will pay for the experimental treatment?

- Will I be reimbursed for other expenses?

- What type of long-term follow-up care is part of this study?

- How will I know that the experimental treatment is working?

- Will results of the trials be provided to me?

Risks and Benefits

There are lots of good reasons to participate in a clinical trial. They give you access to the latest medical treatments and the opportunity to get expert medical care at leading health-care facilities. You'll also be helping others by contributing to medical research.

Of course, there are risks, too. These treatments are still in the testing phase. They may or may not work, and they may very well have unexpected side effects. And if you're in a trial that is testing medications, you may be given a placebo (a pill with inactive ingredients), which means you won't get the drug at all.

Choosing whether you should participate is a very personal decision. It might be helpful to talk it over with your family, friends, and health-care providers, too. The more you know before you sign up, the better. And also know you can resign from a trial at any time.

The Least You Need to Know

- Stem cell research and treatments show promise in treating some back conditions.
- There are lots of different clinical trials looking for candidates to test new back pain medicines and treatments.
- Clinical trials carry risks and benefits.

Meet Your Health-Care Providers

As you'll soon discover in these pages, it takes a village to address your back pain. And with the tips and information here, you'll have the insights to create the best team for your needs. Learn what to look for in good doctors with questions you should ask as well as what questions they should ask you!

You'll learn more about the different kinds of doctors and other health-care professionals who treat back pain and how they've been educated. You might be surprised to learn that some alternative health-care professionals study as long or longer than some conventional medical doctors.

Of course, diagnostic tests will be a part of your back-care journey. You'll learn about the different types of tests and what they reveal. Being informed helps you make more informed health-care choices. This part will help you do just that.

Creating Healing Partnerships

In This Chapter

- Deciding on the best health-care providers for you
- Determining ways to include or exclude providers
- Gathering information and preparing for first visits

It takes a village, the old cliché says. And it could very well take a team of providers to help you through your acute or chronic back pain. You are the chief in this village and you get to decide who's in and who's out. With this authority comes the challenge of making a decision of who to hire. Lots of people are going to want the job. You need to sift carefully through the candidates and prepare yourself for the journey.

Finally, this is your back and your body. A proactive, take-charge attitude will empower you and your decision-making process. Healing is more an art than a science. Different health-care providers have different approaches. Patients' needs vary. Doctor's aren't mind readers or magicians. You have to communicate (and so do they) to get the best care. That's why knowing what you want and need in a provider will help you assemble the right team for you.

Finding Good Health-Care Providers

Some people spend more time researching major purchases such as cars than they do looking into their health-care providers. Truth be told, it can be easier to look into cars than physicians. Many online resources and detailed reports are dedicated to reviewing vehicles, but not so many resources are available for evaluating physicians. And it can also be a little intimidating to ask doctors questions face to face. But you can and should know about the qualifications and experience of people who are treating you. Good physicians really don't mind. Let these tips guide you in looking for everyone who might be on your team, be they medical doctors, physical therapists, or acupuncturists.

> **BODY WISE**
>
> The best medical centers attract among the best medical professionals. Your community's most respected hospital is a good place to look for health-care providers.

Recommendations

The best place to start is recommendations from your primary care physician. If you don't already have one, you need to get one, because your primary care provider should be your first stop. In your search for primary care doctors and other health-care providers, seek recommendations from family, friends, and coworkers. Online communities such as Facebook make this wonderfully easy these days. Use your social networks to get referrals and advice. Ask at work, at church, and at family gatherings. Find out what people like or what they don't like in their providers, and what they'd do differently if they saw this provider again.

Someone who has been to myriad specialists and had bad outcomes may not be the best source from whom to gain referrals. Sure, you can learn from his or her mistakes, but it's more efficient to search for those in your social network who have had a back problem similar to yours and had it treated successfully.

WATCH YOUR BACK

What makes a good doctor? There's an old saying in medicine: to get busy in your practice, either advertise or take good care of patients. These alternatives are not mutually exclusive, but for the most part, good physicians do not need to advertise. If you read reviews of some of the most highly advertised physicians, you will find many disgruntled patients. Those physicians keep busy by bringing new patients in the door to replace the unhappy ones. Also, keep in mind that people, including doctors, can say anything they want about themselves. Some claim they are world-renowned experts, but they are really self-promoted, self-proclaimed World Wide Web experts. We highly recommend you check facts and backgrounds.

Create a list that will help you filter what you want and don't want in a provider. The National Institutes of Health recommends you think about these questions:

- Do you prefer a male or female doctor?

- Do you prefer a younger doctor or an older doctor?

- Where is the doctor's office? Is it easy for you to get to? What's the parking situation?

- Is the doctor part of a group or is he or she a solo practitioner?

- If he or she is a solo practitioner, who covers for the doctor when he or she is away?

- Can you ask questions via phone or e-mail? Is there a charge for this?

- What hours and days do they see patients? How far in advance do you have to make an appointment?

- Does he or she accept your health insurance?

- What hospital(s) is the doctor affiliated with?

Add to this list anything that is important to you. As you'll find out in the next chapter, a primary care or internist will be your first step in getting medical care for your back, so it's crucial to have this type of doctor and to have a good relationship with that person. It takes time to research and establish a rapport with anyone, including a doctor. Think of it like dating: some people are good matches for you, but some aren't. You need someone whose style is a fit for you. You can sometimes weed people out quickly before you even meet them because you have parameters (such as those in the preceding list). Sometimes you'll only know for sure after you've had a few visits with that person.

WATCH YOUR BACK

If a physician or group claims to be the only one offering a certain treatment, beware. If the treatment is so great, why isn't anyone else doing it? Physicians have to complete up to 100 hours of continuing medical education a year. There are no procedures in spine surgery so groundbreaking or so difficult that only a select few can offer them. Most websites that make such grandiose claims are misleading.

Credentials

Of course, medical doctors are licensed. You can check with your state's medical board to ensure that your doctor's license is in good standing. In most states, chiropractors, physical therapists, acupuncturists, and massage therapists must also be licensed and/or certified. We've listed organizations that can help you find out more about a health-care provider and the requirements of the provider's field of expertise.

If the name of the practice contains the word "institute," be aware that this is now a trendy marketing term in the spine care field. Very few "institutes" deserve the title, and those that do are affiliated with a respected teaching hospital and carry out extensive research. Likewise, although the terms "minimally invasive," "laser," "endoscopic," and "arthroscopic" have their place, they are now industry buzzwords, too. Companies pay a lot of money to search engines to use these words and come up at the top of search queries.

Check certification status with the American Board of Medical Specialties (ABMS), which oversees 24 specialty boards (www.abms. org), and at websites such as HealthGrades.com and vitals.com. The governing body of certification is important. There are many "boards" that have no valid affiliation or criteria for screening. A lot of patients have fallen victim to dentists and surgeons who are "board-certified" in plastic surgery after a weekend course.

You can also verify the certifying board with the ABMS. For example, the lofty-sounding American Academy of Neurological and Orthopaedic Surgeons is *not* recognized by the ABMS. To drive the point home, consider that the American Board of Cosmetic Surgery and the American Board of Cosmetic Facial Surgery are also not recognized by the ABMS. The ABMS recognizes plastic surgery as a separate and distinct medical specialty, and has empowered its component organization, the American Board of Plastic Surgery, to establish criteria for training and certification. The other boards mentioned have very little criteria for membership other than the fee required to print the certificate.

Don't be shy about asking questions when you call a provider's office. The provider's staff may know much of these details or they should be able to tell how to find out more. Some of this information is available online. Or you can ask for their resumé or curriculum vitae (basically a longer document with more details than a resumé). Here are a few key things you'll want to know:

- What is the provider's educational background?

- Is the provider board-certified in his or her specialty?

- How long has the provider been in practice? How long has he or she been practicing in this specialty?

- What percentage of the provider's patients are treated for back problems?

- Does the provider believe in alternative or complementary care?

Medical professionals should be board-certified in their specialty. If you see the term "board-eligible," it means that they have not completed their credentialing. Those who are actually certified typically have more experience and have demonstrated that knowledge.

Certifications for other health specialties vary widely. The association websites generally have certification requirements. The more study hours, continuing education requirements, and testing, the better. You definitely want providers who keep their skills and update their knowledge through continuing education. This is as true for a massage therapist as it is for a physician.

The following sites are among the most relevant to your search for back pain–related health-care providers. You can search for providers or look up providers to check their backgrounds.

- **Acupuncturists (www.medicalacupuncture.org):** The American Academy of Medical Acupuncture lists medical doctors who also do acupuncture.

- **Chiropractors (www.acatoday.org):** The American Chiropractic Association is the world's largest professional association representing doctors of chiropractic medicine.

- **Massage therapists (www.amtamassage.org):** The largest organization representing massage therapists is the American Massage Therapy Association.

- **Primary care and other providers (www.ama-assn.org):** The American Medical Association (AMA) is the nation's largest medical society. You can search for medical professionals of all kinds. The results include those who are not AMA members.

- **Neurosurgeons (www.neurosurgerytoday.org):** The American Academy of Neurological Surgeons has a public site where you can search for board-certified surgeons.

- **Orthopedists (www.aaos.org):** You'll find orthopedic (bone) specialists at American Academy of Orthopedic Surgeons.

- **Osteopaths (www.osteopathic.org):** The American Osteopathic Association is the primary certifying body for doctors of osteopathy.

- **Physical therapists (www.apta.org):** The American Physical Therapy Association is the main membership organization that represents physical therapists and promotes physical therapy.

After you narrow down your search, go through your filtering list and delete those items that are nice-to-haves but not need-to-haves. This should help you reduce your list of potential providers to just a few so you can move forward with this process.

Questions and Answers

There are some key questions to ask your health-care provider, and some that your provider should ask you. You might have to make an appointment to discuss these, but it's well worth the investment. When you call the provider's office, explain that you want an appointment to find out whether the provider is a good fit for you. The appointment can be used for a quick information interview or as part of an initial exam, but let the provider's office know you want time to ask questions.

Front-desk personnel might be able to answer some of your questions, or the provider might be willing to talk to you for a few minutes.

What You Should Ask Your Health-Care Provider

If you know the cause of your back problem, ask specifically whether the provider treats that cause, what he or she has done to treat it, and common complications with respect to your back problem. Likewise, if you are considering a procedure, ask whether you can talk with other patients the doctor has treated. Does the provider have a preventive approach to health care? If so, what does that approach consist of?

Finally, if you have a complicated medical condition—and some back situations certainly are—you might want to bring someone with you to your appointment. Ask how the provider feels about that.

Find out whether the provider will give you written instructions and if he or she has any patient care brochures or aids to help you better understand your condition. Patient education is critical when it comes to back care. Providers, especially doctors, don't have a ton of time to teach you all you need to know. But they can and should point you in the right direction with respect to your specific case. Books, brochures, instructional aids, and even videos are some of the materials health-care providers may have on hand or they can tell you where you can get them.

BODY WISE

After your initial visit, evaluate it according to your filtering questions. And write down your answers. Were you comfortable? Did you get to ask all your questions without feeling rushed? Did you understand the answers to your questions? Do you feel confident about this person's ability to treat you? Do you trust the provider? If you have questions, does the provider's office call you back? Ask a question of the office and see whether you actually get a reply. If you don't, find a new doctor. Chances are if the provider's office doesn't provide good patient service before you're a patient, things won't change afterward when you become one.

Finally, good providers will admit when they don't have an answer to your question. The best providers will help you find the answers you seek by referring you to another provider or where you can get more information.

What Your Health-Care Provider Should Ask You

Run for the hills if any doctor suggests a treatment plan or medication before doing a thorough evaluation. The evaluation should include physical tests as well as extensive questions about your condition. Your doctor (and other health-care providers) should want to know how long you've had the problem, what you've done about it, what has helped, and what has made matters worse; they should ask specifics of how your pain feels, and how this problem affects your daily life and the work that you do.

Physically, the provider should want to look at and touch your back and see your posture in several positions (sitting, lying down, walking, sleeping). Be honest about all your answers and responses to the physical tests. If you have to have a few drinks to relieve the pain, tell your doctor. This isn't the time to be stoic. It's the time to be clear about how and what you feel both emotionally and physically.

Preparing for Your Visit

If this is your first visit to this provider, expect to fill out a new patient form. It's a good idea to document the following and keep either in your pain journal (remember that from Chapter 2?) or place it in your health records file. Take this information with you to your appointment.

- Your current health history. What is the nature of your problem, what triggered it, when, and what you've done about it. Again, your pain journal will be a huge help here.

- Your family history. Know how parents, grandparents, aunts, and uncles died. This is especially important if they died young. And if back/spine issues run in the family, this is significant for the provider to know.

- A current list of medicines, including over-the-counter medicines and any supplements. Tell your doctor about any allergies. You can also take any medications with you to show the doctor. However, a well-organized list is better. In fact, everyone should carry an up-to-date medication history in case of an emergency situation.

A record of procedures and surgeries, including dates, outcomes, the name of the hospital or clinic where it was performed, and the name of the health-care provider who performed it.

Bring a Cheat Sheet, Take Notes, and Bring a Friend

It's common to be nervous and a little intimidated. That's why taking a note pad (or your pain journal) can help you remember what you want the provider to know, and it's also a place for you to make notes. This is the school of life for your body. It's okay to reference notes, and cheat sheets are fine in this school! If you feel like you want a friend to be with you, take one. They can help you communicate with your provider and they can be invaluable in helping you remember key points about the visit.

The best patients are willing to share their health and personal histories and are willing to speak up if they don't understand something or if something hasn't worked. They're also the ones who are likely to get the best care.

Finally, have realistic expectations. Although many patients get great relief at different steps along the way, some do not. The cure for lower back pain has been and likely always will be elusive. If any practitioner guarantees you a cure with his or her treatment, run, don't walk, away. For some patients, back pain, much like hypertension and diabetes, has no cure, only treatments.

The Least You Need to Know

- Know your provider's credentials and educational background.
- Get referrals but also create a list that helps you filter what you do want and don't want in a provider.
- Being honest in your communications gets you better health care.
- Doctors and providers should ask lots of questions about your condition and also do a physical evaluation.

Conventional Medical Doctors and Common Tests

In This Chapter

- The reasons your primary care doctor is your first stop in diagnosing and treating back pain
- Tests that assess your physical, neurological, and bone condition
- Medical specialists who diagnose and treat back pain

You've been patient. You've waited a couple of weeks and, even though your back pain hasn't gotten any worse, it sure hasn't gotten any better. Or maybe it has gotten steadily worse even after trying over-the-counter meds and alternative treatments such as massage.

What's next? Who do you call? How and when do you decide to see a specialist? What kinds of tests do doctors do and what do the tests reveal? We'll tell you the answers to those burning questions and more.

In the previous chapter, we gave you strategies for finding a good provider. Here you'll learn more about different docs as well as how they evaluate you.

The Front Line

Believe it or not, the first physician you see for back pain is your primary care doctor. Why? This person has broad knowledge about many illnesses and conditions that can cause back pain. He or she can help narrow down the reasons for your discomfort. And your primary care physician can also rule out (or in) non-spine–related issues, such as bladder or kidney issues and even gynecological problems.

It's best to start from a broad perspective. Otherwise, how do you know whether you should see a bone, nerve, or other specialist? Let your primary care doc guide the process.

> **BODY WISE**
>
> It will be helpful if you know a bit about anatomy and the causes of back pain. Review Chapter 3 in this book and your communications with medical docs will sky rocket.

Another advantage to seeing your primary care physician first is that he or she already has your health history and you have established trust with that person. Good rapport can get you better treatment. You can speak freely and openly about body and mind, which both need to be considered in back pain.

Whether your primary care doc is new to you or you've had a decades-long relationship, the same evaluative rules apply. Your primary care doc should ask lots of questions (when, where, and how it hurts; how long you've had the pain; and how you've treated it). Physical exams should include tests of reflexes, muscle strength, and flexibility. They should also touch your spine and back muscles.

After these initial exams, you may discover that you have what most other people with back pain have: common strain or sprain. As you know, such conditions take time to heal. That's a relief, but you still have to deal with the pain. Your doctor can help the healing process with additional medications, self-help recommendations, and/or a prescription for physical therapy.

If, however, your doctor suspects it may be more than a common strain/sprain, imaging diagnostic tests (X-ray, MRI) may be in your future. Primary care doctors might also order other tests (most likely blood tests) to rule out such things as infections. In the following section, we detail more about the diagnostic tests your primary care physician or other specialists may use to determine the cause of your back pain.

Common Tests

Primary care physicians and specialists use many of the same tests. Always ask why tests are being ordered, what the tests will reveal, how long it will take for the results of the tests to be known, and how you will be informed of the results. Here, we'll help you better understand the purpose of the tests.

Some tests require preparation—for example, not eating or drinking the morning of the test. Be clear about what you need to do and, of course, do it to ensure test accuracy. Likewise, find out whether the test will have any side effects afterward so you can plan your day appropriately.

BODY WISE

High-tech diagnostic tests should come after thorough physical exams. As we've said before, there is normal wear and tear on spine bones and intervertebral discs. These wear patterns show up on tests and may not be the source of pain. For example, simply knowing you have a bulging disc isn't helpful. If the disc isn't pressing on a nerve, it may not be causing pain and may not need treatment.

Physical Tests

Your primary care doctor will administer a physical exam, and if you see a specialist, he or she may very well repeat some of the same tests. They will evaluate such physical factors as your posture, range of motion, reflexes, balance, strength, flexibility, and sensations. Here's some of the commons ways they do it.

The doctor will look at your posture seated, standing, and probably lying down. Be natural and comfortable when you get in these positions. Don't suddenly sit up perfectly straight when your natural position may be a little slouched. To get the care you need, be real.

The doctor can test reflexes by gently tapping your knee (or other body parts) with a small rubber hammer. Testing reflexes reveals what's happening with nerve communication. To test your balance, the doctor may have you stand on one leg—another test that can show how your nervous system is functioning.

Your range of motion and flexibility can be established in several ways. Can you touch your toes from a seated or standing position? How far can you side bend, rotate, and extend backward? All the while, your doctor will rely on your feedback as to when or if the movement causes you pain. Tight muscles can easily be the cause of back pain. And your Rx might simply be to stretch more and take something to help relieve the pain and inflammation.

By touching your back (or *palpating*, in medical jargon), the doctor again is looking for your input. Does it hurt? How so? Your doctor is also looking at your spine to see whether there are any abnormalities.

These physical exams are very much like detective work and it's a process of elimination. Nerve issues can cause pain or loss of sensation. A gentle poke with a paperclip can reveal whether there is such a loss. A lift of a leg that causes pain is a sign of sciatic nerve trouble. Likewise, if reflexes don't respond, there may be an interruption in your nerve pathway. If your pain is worse when you bend forward, that could indicate a problem with intervertebral discs; if it's worse when you bend backward, that could mean spinal stenosis or arthritis in a facet joint. If your pain minimizes after waking, that's an indicator that osteoarthritis may be the culprit.

Physical tests not only help diagnose the potential problem, they also point to which additional tests should come next in the search for the cause of your back pain.

THE BACK AND BEYOND

The combination of nerves and muscles working together is called the neuromuscular system. When you want your body to move, the brain sends an electrical signal through your motor nerves. When the signal reaches muscle fibers, chemical messengers (neurotransmitters) cause a chain reaction that stimulates a muscle to move. The activity along the neuromuscular pathway can be detected by special machines.

Neurological Tests

Physical neurological tests include evaluating your balance, coordination, reflexes, and muscle strength. If an oddity is discovered, the following neurological tests can help determine whether it's a nerve-related condition. Typically, a specialist such as a physiatrist or neurologist (see the section "The Medical Specialists" later in this chapter) will order neurological tests.

Electromyography (EMG) is often combined with nerve condition studies such as a nerve conduction study (NCS) test. These tests evaluate your *peripheral nervous system (PNS)*. An EMG looks at the electrical activity of your nerves and muscles. An NCS monitors the speed at which electrical signals travel through a nerve. You don't have to do anything to prepare for these tests, but the procedures can be a bit uncomfortable for reasons that will soon become obvious.

DEFINITIONS

Nerves that are outside the spinal canal and cranium are referred to as peripheral and belong to the **peripheral nervous system (PNS).** The PNS includes both sensory and motor nerves. Sensory nerves, as the term implies, enable sensation, such as feeling someone tickle you, or knowing if something is hot, cold, wet, dry, sharp, or soft. Motor nerves, on the other hand, carry out automatic functions (such as breathing and circulation) and also enable voluntary muscle movements (walking, lifting objects, scratching your nose, and so on).

To conduct an EMG, a specialist inserts fine needles into your muscles. The needles are hooked up to an EMG machine that detects and records electrical patterns that nerves produce. An EMG thus assesses the health of your muscles and the nerves that supply them.

During an EMG test, you'll be asked to move a body part, such as to lift your arm. The response patterns of your nerves show up as wavelengths on a special scope and can also be heard through speakers. The nerve generates signals that actually sound like radio static. The test shows how your muscles and nerves respond to a stimulus (such as your brain telling you to lift your arm). After the test, you might have some bruising or tenderness where the needles were inserted, but other than that, there are no side effects.

Nerve conduction studies use two sets of electrodes, similar to electrocardiogram patches, which are placed on your chest to test heart function. In nerve conduction studies, the electrodes are adhered to the skin over muscles (no needles are used). With a mild electrical shock, one electrode stimulates a nerve that runs to a particular muscle. The second electrode measures the speed at which impulses travel through the nerve. The result of the test reveals how well the nerve is functioning. Sometimes it can reveal a pinched nerve outside of the back or some other neurological problem. The shocks can be uncomfortable but are rarely painful. This test has no side effects once they stop zapping you.

Imaging Tests

A variety of tests can show what's going on with your bones and soft tissues. Again, these tests are not your first point of evaluation. They come later in the process, because common age-related abnormalities in soft tissues and bones show up in imaging tests but may not be the cause of pain, and because some of these tests are very expensive and may not change the course of treatment. For example, osteoarthritis has treatment methods that can be tried without major concern about side effects. If all indications are that the patient has arthritis, why not treat the symptoms accordingly? Tests are best when there are still questions about what is happening or to confirm status when contemplating surgery.

Common X-rays show issues affecting bones and their structure, such as a vertebral fracture, infection, or bone tumor. The results are quick and can be on physical film or on a computer screen. It's the same painless procedure you've probably experienced many times in the dentist's chair, only this time, they're taking pictures of your back.

Dynamic X-rays are used to evaluate motion of the spine. Typically they are taken at each extreme of bending. The bending may be forward and backward (flexion and extension) or side to side (lateral bending). These tests can show spinal instability during movement.

Computerized tomography (CT), also known as a computed axial tomography (CAT scan), is an advancement of the common X-ray in that it shows bones in great detail. It also provides basic information about soft tissue (muscles, tendons, discs). It's good for verifying whether an intervertebral disc rupture, spinal stenosis, or damaged vertebra is the culprit in back pain. It's a fast and painless option. However, it does not show nerves very well. Orthopedic specialists, which we'll discuss shortly, often use this type of scan when a patient has had an accident or fall, as it shows more detail than an ordinary X-ray.

Magnetic resonance imaging (MRI) is similar to an X-ray but uses a powerful magnetic field and radio waves (instead of radiation), which are translated into three-dimensional computer images of your spine and soft tissues. The images are quite detailed and show the positioning of vertebrae, discs, nerve roots, and the spinal cord. MRIs are typically ordered for surgical reasons, as it will help surgeons see the specific problem areas (where nerves are being pinched). The machines are expensive and so are the tests, generally ranging from $1,000 to $2,000, so make sure you find out in advance whether your insurance will cover such a test.

THE BACK AND BEYOND

Contrast dyes are sometimes used with MRIs or CT scans. Two tests that use dyes are discography and myelography. As the name implies, greater contrast between structures can be seen when these dyes are introduced into the body. For example, a contrast agent can enhance the view of an intervertebral disc and surrounding structures. For spine imaging, the dye is injected. If you have any allergies, definitely tell your doctor before a contrast dye is given to you.

MRI scans involve your whole body being placed in a large cylinder. It's noisy and narrow and you stay still in there for a good 30 minutes or more. If you're claustrophobic (and it's hard not to be in one of those things), your doctor may give you a mild anti-anxiety medication. Also, because a giant magnet is involved, MRIs can't be performed on anyone who has metal in his or her body, such as shrapnel, a pacemaker, or certain aneurysm clips.

Discography is used to test whether a disc is the source of your pain. A special contrast dye is injected into a spinal disc thought to be causing lower back pain. If the injection triggers your pain, that disc may be a source of your problem. If it doesn't reproduce the pain, the disc is not the source of pain. Often, a CT scan is done after the injection of this dye. The dye fills the disc and can illustrate damaged areas in the disc. Doctors sometimes order discographies for patients who are considering surgery for a suspected disc problem. The injection can be painful as the needle goes through muscle and other tissue to get to the disc. The other risks involve infection, bleeding, and worsening of symptoms.

A myelography is similar to discography in that a contrast dye is used. In this case, the dye is injected into the spinal canal and images are taken via a fluoroscope, a special X-ray machine that shows real-time moving images. A CT scan may also be taken. The procedure shows whether there is nerve compression in the spinal canal. The injection itself can be painful. In a small number of cases, spinal fluid might leak out of the pinhole at the site of the dye injection. The result is a headache that can last for a couple of days. Myelograms are often done on patients who cannot have an MRI because they have a metal implant or metal screws in their back.

Bone scans diagnose the presence of tumors, infections, fractures, or other bone disorders. Radioactive material is injected into the bloodstream and absorbed by the bones. It takes a couple of hours for the material to make its way to the bones, after which an image is scanned by a special machine. Radioactive material collects in areas where there is a problem and shows up as a hot spot on the image. Injecting radioactivity sounds like a scary prospect, but the amounts used are very small—about the same amount you'd get from a couple of X-rays.

The Medical Specialists

Becoming a doctor requires four years of pre-med and four years of medical school (two in the classroom, two in a clinical setting). After getting their degree as a medical doctor or osteopath, graduates apply for residency. At this point, they are degreed medical doctors practicing on real patients (typically in a hospital setting), but they are still considered students in training and are supervised by an attending physician. Residency is like a paid internship. Most states require at least a year of residency training, after which doctors are licensed to practice medicine in that state. This first year of residency is typically called an internship.

BODY WISE

In a hospital, especially a teaching hospital, you may be treated by a resident doctor (who is still in training). If your situation is complicated, or you feel unsure about the treatment you're receiving, ask to see the attending physician, who has completed his or her training and is fully licensed. If you're undergoing surgery, understand that residents may be involved. If so, they are closely supervised by the attending physician, an ethical and legal requirement. A resident involved in your case will have a particular interest in your well-being since it reflects on them. It's like having a second doctor involved, and often they will take more time with you than the attending physician. If you're uncomfortable with the resident actually performing the procedure, request that the attending physician do it while the other watches.

Becoming a medical specialist requires many more years of training. For example, an internist (an internal medicine specialist, not an intern) studies another three years. A neurosurgeon typically trains for another seven years (that's in addition to the eight years already spent in pre-med and medical school). Specialists aren't required to be board-certified, but it's worth looking for a specialist who has undergone board-specific training.

Finally, some physicians undergo additional training beyond residency. This is called a fellowship. It is more specialized, similar to an apprenticeship. Orthopedic surgeons typically do these to get additional training in spine surgery. Neurosurgeons are qualified to operate on the spine without doing a fellowship.

The educational process never really ends for any physician. They have to keep up to date with new medicines, procedures, and treatment options, and, fortunately, continuing medical education is required. License renewals vary by state. In most states, physicians must keep and submit their continuing medical education (CME) credits every year or two.

Pain-Management Physicians

The American Board of Medical Specialties says that a pain-management specialist should be an M.D. with board certification in at least one of the following specialties: anesthesiology, physical rehabilitation, psychiatry, or neurology. Pain-management specialists help people reduce pain and regain quality of life. You might be referred to a pain-management specialist after back surgery or if your back pain has become chronic or is recurring. The phrase "it takes a village" applies here. Patients who are in severe and/or chronic pain need to manage it from several angles: physically, psychologically, and medically. That's why patients will have a pain-management team composed of several disciplines.

Neurologists and Orthopedists

Neurologists specialize in nonsurgical treatment of both the peripheral and central nervous system (brain and spinal cord). They help diagnose causes of pain, including pinched nerves. In addition, they treat patients with fibromyalgia, seizures, strokes, and Alzheimer's Disease.

Orthopedists focus on issues related to muscles and bones, referred to in medical lingo as the musculoskeletal system. They treat skeletal bones, including the spine, and their tissues (muscles, tendons, and ligaments). Some focus more on scoliosis or pain caused by problems in the hip joint. You'll also see this specialty spelled as *orthopaedics*.

Physiatrists

Physiatrists specialize in physical medicine, meaning they help people who are physically impaired. The field expanded after World War II when soldiers returned with physical injuries. Patients with back problems are referred to physiatrists to help them get moving again. Physiatrists prescribe medications, therapeutic exercise with a physical therapist, assistive devices (such as canes), and orthotics (braces). Physiatrists might also be called physical medicine or rehab specialists.

Training to become a physiatrist is less extensive than that of the other specialties mentioned, but can last a decade or longer if the candidate plans to subspecialize in areas such as neuromuscular medicine or traumatic brain injury.

Rheumatologists

You might be familiar with a rheumatologist as a doctor who treats people with arthritis. These professionals' scope of practice is broader, however, as they treat painful disorders of the joints and soft tissues (muscles, tendons, connective tissue) and also autoimmune diseases. Ankylosing spondylitis is a type of chronic and progressive arthritis of the spine, which in severe forms causes a bent-forward position. It is also an autoimmune disease. Other back issues that a rheumatologist might treat include osteoporosis and fibromyalgia. Like the other specialists mentioned here, rheumatologists train for several years beyond their initial degree of medical doctor.

BODY WISE

Arthritis is an umbrella term used to describe more than 100 different conditions that affect joints and tissues of the musculoskeletal system. Conditions that affect soft tissues around the joint include tendonitis and bursitis; those that affect the bone include osteoarthritis and spinal stenosis.

The Surgeons

As if a decade of education weren't enough, another several years of training are required to become a surgeon. When it comes to spine surgery, you'll be referred to either a neurosurgeon or an orthopedic surgeon. They perform many of the same surgeries for spine conditions.

THE BACK AND BEYOND

If you're facing surgery, you may be surprised to learn that neurosurgeons do more spine surgery than surgeons from any other specialty. Although they operate on the entire neuroaxis (brain, spinal cord, and nerves), most of their work involves the spine. Neurosurgeons also perform peripheral nerve surgery and can treat pinched nerves outside of the spine. They also treat spinal-cord tumors, nerve tumors, spina bifida, and other neural tube defects.

Neurosurgeons

Neurosurgeons specialize in surgical treatments of the nervous system. They treat ruptured disks, sciatica, and other sources of lower back pain. In addition to treating and diagnosing back and neck issues, neurosurgeons may see people with brain injuries and other nervous system conditions such as aneurysms and tumors. Aside from neurosurgeons' treatment of brain conditions, however, their specialty has tremendous overlap with orthopedists in treating spine conditions.

Orthopedic Surgeons

Orthopedic surgeons who specialize in the spine treat herniated and degenerated discs, stenosis, fractures, and instability much like neurosurgeons. Some orthopedic surgeons also perform peripheral nerve surgery. However, as bone specialists, they also focus more on hip joints, sacroiliac disease, and arthritic causes of back pain. Most scoliosis (deformity) surgery is still done by orthopedic surgeons.

For more on the types of surgeries available for back pain, see Chapter 9.

The Least You Need to Know

- The first medical doctor to see for your back should be your primary care doctor.
- Common in-office physical tests include those that analyze your balance, flexibility, muscle strength, and reflexes.
- Diagnostic tests such as MRIs and CT scans should come after physical tests.
- A variety of medical specialists treat back pain. Your primary care doc will refer you to the right one.

Complementary and Alternative Care Providers

In This Chapter

- CAM therapies you're most likely to encounter for back pain
- How CAM providers are educated
- What to look for in CAM providers
- State regulation and licensing requirements

"First, do no harm," is a fundamental principle taught in medical school. We believe the same holds true for complementary and alternative providers as well. Unlike conventional medicine however, complementary and alternative medicine (CAM) isn't as regulated, although many states do require licensing for some practices. This doesn't make such providers less valuable, but because there's less accountability, it does make it easier for those who are unscrupulous to make promises they can't keep. Your diligence in selecting providers will help weed out potential charlatans.

As you'll read here, CAM providers can be quite well trained and educated. According to the National Institute of Complementary and Alternative Medicine, a branch of the National Institutes of Health, back pain is the number one reason that people seek CAM therapies.

In this chapter, we cover those CAM therapy providers that you are most likely to encounter in your search for back pain relief. We shed light on how these providers are typically educated and what you should look for in terms of experience and credentials.

Complementary Care Providers

In general, CAM practitioners ask that patients participate in the healing process. They may recommend exercises or self-treatments. Some practitioners shun pharmaceuticals, believing that drugs mask symptoms and thwart the body's innate ability to heal itself. We believe that conventional medicines and treatments combined with CAM therapies can work well for many people. Some people may find relief solely through an alternative therapy, and that's great, too.

As a final note, a reminder about the difference between alternative and complementary providers: Alternative generally means therapies that are used in place of conventional medicine; complementary means therapies that are used in addition to conventional medicine. Depending on your doctor's philosophy, he or she may recommend therapies from either of these camps.

WATCH YOUR BACK

Beware of anyone who promises to cure your back pain or asks you to commit up front to a series of treatments. It's fine to know how many sessions the provider believes you'll need to find relief, but avoid purchasing a package up front until you've had a session or two.

The conventional medicine community has embraced and recommended a number of CAM therapies for which there is scientific evidence. In the medical world, this is referred to as evidence-based medicine. The most common CAM therapies physicians recommend for back pain are acupuncture, chiropractic manipulation, and massage therapy. All three treatments have scientific proof that they can help relieve back pain.

As we've previously mentioned, a new branch of medicine called integrative medicine endorses many CAM practices and includes them within the branch's own scopes of practice. Medical centers that include integrative medicine departments have such providers as massage therapists, chiropractic doctors, and acupuncturists on their staffs. We've covered the specifics on what to expect from these therapies in Chapter 7. Here's the skinny on the providers.

Acupuncturists

The American Academy of Physician Acupuncturists (AAPA) is an organization for medical doctors who practice acupuncture. The AAPA refers to their practice as medical acupuncture. To be a full member of this organization, the practitioner must have a current medical license as a medical doctor or doctor of osteopathy; have completed 220 hours of acupuncture training; and have two years of experience as a medical acupuncturist.

THE BACK AND BEYOND

The AAPA was founded in 1987 by a group of physicians who were graduates of the Medical Acupuncture for Physicians training programs sponsored by University Extension, UCLA School of Medicine. AAPA represents physician members in the United States and Canada.

Acupuncture training programs vary. The one offered for physicians through Harvard Medical School is a nine-month program offering 300 credit hours. For those who are not medical doctors, the more rigorous schools require three to four years of training (about 3,000 hours). A comprehensive training program includes a thorough understanding of traditional Chinese medicine, which includes acupuncture, anatomy, herbal medicine, and advanced needling techniques. Sadly, there are also online courses that offer certificates of completion, enabling unqualified persons to actually practice.

Before allowing anyone to stick needles in you, ask about his or her education in terms of years and hours of schooling, clinical/practical experience, and state licensing. Also ask about their experience in treating patients with back pain and what you should expect in terms of pain relief.

Acupuncture is regulated state by state. Some don't require any licenses; others require a certification from the National Certification Commission for Acupuncture and Oriental Medicine (NCCAOM). This organization tests individuals and requires continuing education and a license renewal every four years. For information on what your state requires, see the organization's website at www.nccaom.org.

Chiropractors

Chiropractic is the largest, most regulated of the CAM professions. It is the third-largest doctoral-level health-care profession after conventional medicine and dentistry. Chiropractic is state-regulated and licensed. All states require a license to practice.

The Council on Chiropractic Education, an agency certified by the U.S. Department of Education, is the accrediting body for chiropractic colleges in the United States. Generally, to qualify for admission into an accredited chiropractor training program, the candidate must have a few years of undergraduate college credit, mostly in sciences.

The chiropractor program itself is a four-year program requiring both classroom and clinical work. Studies include anatomy, physiology, microbiology, biochemistry, pathology, nutrition, and hands-on work with patients. Graduates receive a doctor of chiropractic degree, after which they are eligible to sit for a state licensing exam.

All states require chiropractic doctors to be licensed. Each state's requirements vary. Most require at least two years of education (beyond undergrad) and increasingly that requirement is becoming four years. National board examinations for licensing include a mock patient encounter. To maintain their licenses, chiropractors in most states are required to earn annual continuing education credits. For more information, go to the American Chiropractic Association website at www.acatoday.org.

> **THE BACK AND BEYOND**
>
> The first chiropractic adjustment was performed in 1895 by David Daniel Palmer, the man who created the practice. He coined the term *chiropractic*, which comes from the Greek words *cheir* (hand) and *praktos* (done)—that is, *done by hand*.

Massage Therapists

Compared to the preceding types of health-care providers, becoming a massage therapist requires far less schooling. To get the basic certification or diploma, students learn anatomy, business practices, and ethics, and, of course, practice hands-on techniques. Credible programs require at least 500 hours of training and take about a year to complete. Typically, those who go through a clinical massage therapy program get more in-depth training. Usually, a state board or an accredited independent agency such as the Commission on Massage Therapy Accreditation (COMTA) approves massage training programs. Many states require formal training and licensure in order to practice massage therapy.

WATCH YOUR BACK

Know the difference between a certified and a licensed massage therapist. When it comes to massage, certification means that someone successfully passed a training program. It could be a great program or a mediocre one. Certification is voluntary. Licensure is a requirement by the state and has rigorous standards and testing procedures that a massage therapist must pass to practice in a given state.

Look for massage therapists who attended schools with COMTA accreditation, have at least 500 hours of schooling, and participate in continuing education. Also, membership in a credible professional association shows professionalism. The American Massage Therapy Association is the largest such nonprofit association.

The majority of states do require licensing and passing of a national exam, typically through the National Certification Board for Therapeutic Massage and Bodywork (NCBTMB). Most states also require that massage therapists participate in continuing education and carry malpractice insurance. To find out your state's requirements, go to www.massageregister.com/massage-license-requirements.

THE BACK AND BEYOND

Only a few states do not require massage therapists to be licensed: Alaska, Idaho, Kansas, Minnesota, Montana, Oklahoma, Vermont, and Wyoming. Massage therapy may be regulated at the local level in these states. Laws often change, however, so it is best to check information on licensing, certification, and accreditation on a state-by-state basis.

Understand that medical massage therapy is separate from conventional massage therapy. Some states even have special certification for the medical variety. Both are beneficial, but you're not likely to have insurance coverage for lavender-infused massage oil and cucumber water while lounging around in a white fluffy robe listening to Enya.

Alternative Medicine Providers

Here we get into murkier waters with respect to state requirements. Few if any laws exist to regulate the following practices. Again, lack of regulation doesn't make these practices less credible, it just invites the unscrupulous to practice more freely. And health claims of cures can be more routinely bandied about without evidence.

Use your instincts. Talk to providers about their methodology and experience with back pain. Here are the basics on how these providers get educated in their fields.

Naturopaths

To become a qualified naturopath is similar to becoming a medical doctor. These are highly educated practitioners. A Bachelor's degree is required for entrance into naturopathic school. Naturopathic medical students study the same medical curriculum as conventional medical students. Clinical hours working directly with patients (under the supervision of a licensed naturopathic physician [ND]) is also a part of their education.

THE BACK AND BEYOND

National Institutes of Health researchers found that a naturopathic approach (acupuncture, exercise, and relaxation training) for treating lower back pain in warehouse workers was more cost-effective than the employer's usual patient education program. The outcomes included better health-related quality of life, less absenteeism, and lower costs for other treatments and pain medication.

In naturopathy, the objective is to treat the whole person (not just a disease) and to improve a person's overall well-being. Therefore, naturopathic studies emphasize holistic and nontoxic therapies such as clinical nutrition, acupuncture, homeopathy, and herbal medicine. To help coach people through lifestyle changes, naturopaths also study psychology and counseling strategies.

According to the Association of Accredited Natural Medical Colleges, there are six fundamental principles of naturopathic medicine:

1. **First, do no harm:** Utilize the most natural, least invasive, and least toxic therapies.

2. **The healing power of nature:** Trust in the body's inherent wisdom to heal itself.

3. **Identify and treat the causes:** Look beyond the symptoms to the underlying cause.

4. **Doctor as teacher:** Educate patients in the steps to achieving and maintaining health.

5. **Treat the whole person:** View the body as an integrated whole in all its physical and spiritual dimensions.

6. **Prevention:** Focus on overall health, wellness, and disease prevention.

Only 15 states license naturopaths. In those states, a naturopath is considered essentially the same as a primary care doctor. In non-regulated states, look for NDs who have attended a four-year college and participate in continuing education. To find a credentialed doctor and learn more about their scope of practice, see www.naturopathic.org.

BODY WISE

Currently, the following states and territories require naturopaths to be licensed: Alaska, Arizona, California, Connecticut, the District of Columbia, Hawaii, Idaho, Kansas, Maine, Minnesota, Montana, New Hampshire, Oregon, Puerto Rico, Utah, Vermont, the Virgin Islands, and Washington. Regulatory laws do change from year to year. Check with your state licensing board to confirm whether or not a naturopath must be licensed in your state.

Homeopaths

These health-care providers, called homeopathic doctors, generally receive some basic college-level education in anatomy, physiology, pathology, and disease. In addition, they study remedies (homeopathic medicines) and how to diagnose and treat people as individuals. In other words, two people can report the same back pain but receive different remedies. The remedies are specially prepared all-natural diluted plant, animal, or mineral substances. Homeopathic medicines have been recognized since 1796.

> **BODY WISE**
>
> Homeopathic remedies are prepared according to the guidelines of the Homeopathic Pharmacopeia of the United States (HPUS), which was written into law in the Federal Food, Drug, and Cosmetic Act in 1938.

Interest in this field is growing in the United States. Some homeopathy courses are structured specifically for medical doctors who are interested in adding this healing modality to their practice. Homeopathy is included in the course work for naturopaths.

Homeopathy is a recognized practice worldwide. Regulation varies. It is not regulated in the United States but it is in France and Austria. Public health programs in the United Kingdom and Denmark cover homeopathy treatments.

In the United States, schools and their requirements do vary quite a bit. Look for homeopathic doctors who have at least 500 hours of training. And ask about their experience with back pain.

Herbalists

Plants have long been used for healing; they were the first medicines. Today, plants are the foundation of many pharmaceuticals. Herbal medicine continues to be a vital practice in many cultures, especially among the Chinese.

Herbalists are health-care providers who may or may not be associated with traditional Chinese medicine. There are short courses of study lasting about six months and others that require several years of study. The field is not regulated in the United States.

The American Herbalists Guild is the standards-setting body that defines educational guidelines for those seeking a comprehensive education. They recommend practitioners obtain 1,600 hours of study, 400 hours of which should be supervised clinical training. Course work should include basic sciences (anatomy, physiology, biochemistry, pathology, and medical terminology) along with many hours in therapeutic herbalism.

When seeking an herbalist, ask about hours of education and experience treating back pain. To find an herbalist and learn more about the practice, go to www.americanherbalistsguild.com.

Traditional Chinese Medicine Practitioners

Traditional Chinese medicine (TCM) is one of the oldest and most widely used traditional medical systems in the world. It incorporates traditional medicines and therapeutic practices from ancient China. As such, practitioners of TCM may recommend and/or administer acupuncture, traditional Chinese herbs, nutritional guidelines, and/or shiatsu massage. Some may specialize in a therapeutic area such as acupuncture or traditional Chinese herbs.

Most programs are Master's programs requiring fours years of full-time study (about 3,000 hours), which includes clinical training. Schools carrying accreditation from the Accreditation Commission for Acupuncture and Oriental Medicine (ACAOM) are considered among the best. Some schools offer clinical courses for M.D.s who want to integrate TCM into their scope of practice.

Most states license acupuncture, but states vary in their regulation of TCM therapies. Almost all licensing states require completion of the National Certification Commission for Acupuncture and Oriental Medicine (NCCAOM) written exam; some states also require a practical exam.

Finally, remember to communicate among your providers. If you are on a blood thinner or have a bleeding disorder, make sure to inform all of your team what you are taking. Don't be shy. Many herbal remedies can interact with conventional medications in a harmful way.

The Least You Need to Know

- CAM practitioners often have levels of education similar to those of conventional medical doctors.

- Some CAM therapies have a long history and come to us from centuries-old healing practices of other countries.

- Regulation of CAM providers varies by state.

- Chiropractic is the most regulated CAM therapy; all states require chiropractors to be licensed.

- Unregulated does not mean unqualified; you need to ask about credentials, education, and licensing to evaluate a provider.

Building a Better Back

Can you do anything to prevent back pain from reoccurring? Yes! We present ideas for how you can improve your back and body every day. From exercises to on-the-job tools and techniques, this part contains a wealth of resources to help you feel better now and later. We also include a chapter about the neck, because neck pain and back pain can so often be notorious companions.

Of course, for many people, physical activity may be limited for a while, and that includes sex. But that doesn't mean you can't get your groove on. We'll provide you with some ideas for keeping your love life alive. This is definitely a chapter to share. Read it, underline it, and use it!

Exercise for a Happy, Healthy Back

14

In This Chapter

- How much and what kind of exercises you need
- Why weight is an issue in back pain
- Seven strategies for successful weight loss and fitness
- How to get more exercise into your day

Hardly a day goes by without a health report citing the value of exercise to our well-being. It helps maintain a healthy spine and it's vital in rehabbing from back pain and injuries. Even those with chronic back pain understand the importance of good physical conditioning. For the majority of people who have common strain/sprain back pain, exercise will help relieve pain and reduce the chances of it reoccurring.

Of course, exercise is no guarantee that your back will never hurt. Sometimes a wrong move or too much exercise can actually cause a problem. But the bottom line is that if you want your body to feel good, you need to exercise it. When you get moving, you'll experience the feel-good benefits for yourself.

Each person's back issue is unique. Consult with your doctors and/or physical therapist before doing any exercises. Here we'll give you an overview of what to do and why and some strategies on how to incorporate physical activity into your life.

How Much Exercise Do You Really Need?

When it comes to exercise, what's the magic number? According to the U.S. Department of Health and Human Services, 30 to 60 minutes a day on most days will help improve strength, increase energy, decrease stress, and help you sleep better, too. All that from exercise! Imagine the profits if someone discovered a pill that could do all that!

WATCH YOUR BACK

Exercising in a pool is a good place to start, as the buoyancy of water helps reduce impact while also providing resistance. Most experts in back pain agree that there is no better exercise for the back than swimming.

Exercise really is the answer for so many things that ail us as a nation: obesity; heart disease; high blood pressure; and, of course, back pain. The fun part is there are many, many ways to get and stay in shape. The key is to find things you enjoy or at least can tolerate until you start feeling the benefits.

Depending on your starting point, it may take some time. And you may have to try different things until you find activities that you enjoy. But truth is, once you get into the routine, you'll feel better physically and mentally. And then, of course, there's the wonderful side effect of looking better, too. Bonus!

BODY WISE

Studies have shown that short bursts of activity can be very beneficial. Have a 15-minute sit-up/push-up/stretch routine in the morning; take a brisk 15-minute walk before lunch; and then have a stroll and easy stretch after dinner—and you've just fit 45 minutes of exercise into your day. Easy!

The problem is, some people hear the word "exercise" and want to run away screaming. Of course, running away would be fine, and the screaming could help your lung capacity, too. But you don't have to be a gym rat to be in good physical condition. Don't even think of it as exercise; instead, just think of daily physical activity. That could be walking your dog, gardening, shoveling snow, or washing the car. The key is moving your body. And for back pain, a few key stretches and muscle strengthening moves should be a part of your routine.

Balanced Muscles for a Healthy Back

Simply put, muscles move and stabilize bones. To do their job effectively, muscles also need to be conditioned in a balanced manner. Most strain/sprain back pain is caused by an imbalance. Either a muscle suddenly got pulled too hard or a repetitive movement pattern caused an imbalance.

If you work at a computer all day and your shoulders and spine roll forward (this is common), the muscles in the front of your body shorten and those in the back are fatigued. That's why it feels so good to stretch backward after sitting all day. You are opening tightened muscles in your chest area.

In addition to stretching, it's really important to strengthen muscles. Better-conditioned abdominals and lower and upper back muscles will help you maintain proper posture. Strong back muscles will help you keep your shoulders more open (so will posture awareness). Balanced muscles and good posture will help prevent fatigue, as well as back and neck pain.

What Kind of Exercise?

For a well-balanced, functional body, we need three types of exercise: aerobic, strength building, and stretching. How you go about those is really up to you, but if you rarely work out, it's smart to invest in a few sessions with a personal trainer or get exercises from your physical therapist. Poor exercise form can create more back problems.

Aerobic exercise increases your heart rate (how fast your pulse is beating), strength builds muscles, and stretching helps you to be more flexible. The trio is a powerful combination for creating a strong and happy back and body for life. We'll give you a taste of some good options to try in the next few chapters.

Why Lose Weight?

Being overweight not only puts excess strain on your back, it overloads your hips, knees, and feet. As you may recall from Chapter 3, most of your body's weight rests in the lower back and hip area. That excess weight puts more pressure on those bones. Losing weight has so many health benefits, but we recognize it's not easy. If it were, we wouldn't have such an obesity problem in this nation and, increasingly, worldwide.

We think the best approach to weight loss is one step at a time. You know the cliché (it may be tired but it's true): successful weight loss requires a lifestyle change. Slowly adopt a few new fitness and food habits and you'll be well on your way. Here are seven strategies to help you be more successful:

1. **Expect to fail.** You're more likely to succeed in changing your behavior if you think of it as learning how to do something new. A natural part of the learning process is failure.

When you learned to ride a bike, you didn't pedal perfectly down the block on the very first try. Chances are you kept at it until riding that bike became second nature. So it is with a healthy lifestyle. At first you don't completely succeed.

2. **Gain emotional perspective.** When you do fail, don't beat yourself up. Instead ask yourself three key questions: What happened? Is there anything you can do about it now? And most importantly, what can you do to prevent it in the future? Everyone falls off the wagon—including high-performing athletes! Don't focus on the negative; instead, analyze yourself, correct the problem, and get back on the wagon as quickly as possible.

3. **Set realistic goals.** Lose 10 pounds in 10 days! Um, no way. Not if you want to keep it off. Instead, go for slow and steady. And don't freak out if you suddenly gain a pound or two. Evaluate over a month's time, not a few day's time.

4. **Break goals into daily actions.** Instead of just saying you want to exercise more, vow to walk for 30 minutes four times a week. Be specific and realistic. And if you can find a goal buddy, partners can motivate each other when the going gets tough.

5. **Think differently.** Sometimes we think that losing weight is about deprivation. We eat well all day, then think, "Gosh darn it, I deserve that gigantic bowl of ice cream!" Healthy eating is about feeling better and getting down to a normal weight. Reward yourself in a nonsabotaging way: music downloads, a movie night, or a new outfit.

6. **Create a supportive environment.** It's easier to have self-control when the cookies and ice cream are still in the grocery store. It's easier to maintain portion control when you don't overload your plate or have large bowls of pasta on the kitchen table. When eating out, especially when ordering pasta, ask for a half order or have the restaurant serve half and put the other portion in a to-go container.

7. **Consider the company you keep.** Studies show that who we eat with affects our behaviors. If your friends overeat and are out of shape, you'll tend to be the same. Conversely, if your friends are physically active and eat wisely, you'll tend to be that way, too. You can't change family and friends overnight, and we're not suggesting that you do. But you can make your health a priority. Again, the buddy system works. It provides mutual support, accountability, and inspiration.

Lunchtime Fitness

Building a stronger, more flexible body needn't take that much time. Fitting a little fitness into a few of your lunch breaks can help. These simple strategies can help you get the most out of your limited lunch hour.

Multitask

Multitasking has its benefits in the office and in the gym. Get maximum benefit from limited time by combining cardiovascular exercise with strength training. For example, hop on a cardio machine for 10 minutes, weight train your upper body for 10 minutes, then stretch. Alternate between upper and lower body weight training each time you work out to get a full-body benefit by the week's end. Entice a coworker to join you. You can brainstorm new ideas and build better professional relationships, too.

No Gym? Bring It In

You don't need a lot of space to exercise efficiently. Get a yoga mat and a resistance band and you've got your own in-office workout. Resistance bands offer an endless array of strength-training and stretching options. They can be done standing, sitting, or lying down. These bands are inexpensive and most come with step-by-step workout routines. Or gather a group and hire a group fitness trainer to come to your worksite.

You can do many exercises without any equipment. Think calisthenics: push-ups, sit-ups, squats, and jumping jacks. Good form, precision, and control are key. Even stepping away from the computer for a few minutes to stretch out your back can help reduce stiffness. A few side stretches, forward bends, and gentle spine twists work wonders.

Active at the Office

What else can you do to add more activity to your workday? Plenty!

- Stand while talking on the telephone.

- Walk down the hall to speak with someone rather than using the telephone or e-mail.

- Get off the elevator a few floors early and take the stairs the rest of the way.

- Participate in or start a weight-loss competition at your company.

- Form a team to raise money for charity events.

- Join a fitness center or Y near your job. Work out before or after work to avoid rush-hour traffic, or drop by for a noon workout.

- Get off the bus a few blocks early and walk the rest of the way to work or home.

- Walk around your building for a break during the workday or during lunch.

The Least You Need to Know

- For maximum benefit from exercise, you need 30 to 60 minutes of activity most days of the week.

- You can break up exercise into short bursts of activity instead of doing it in one longer session.

- You need strength, flexibility, and aerobic exercise for a well-functioning body.

- If you're overweight, losing excess pounds reduces stress on your back.

- To create a healthy lifestyle, you need sound strategies that include acceptance of failure and ways to overcome it.

Lengthen and Strengthen with Pilates

In This Chapter

* Why Pilates is good for your back
* Hallmarks of good instruction
* Important details of this mind-body exercise
* Five core and back strengthening exercises to try

Pilates exercises help you develop long, lean muscles by lengthening and strengthening muscles at the same time. Proper alignment of the spine, breathing, concentration, and awareness are all part of this mind-body discipline. It's an intense, refreshing, and invigorating workout. And you will most certainly work your abs, a lot. You'll find Pilates classes and private sessions in specialized studios, health clubs, and community centers nationwide.

Here we provide tips on finding good instruction and share with you a few back-benefiting moves to try on your own. Of course, these moves may not be ideal for everyone, so be sure to get exercise clearance from your physicians and/or consult with your physical therapist.

It's About Control

Pilates is often described as an intense abdominal workout. It is that and so much more. Perhaps the best definition comes from the man who created this mind-body discipline. Joseph H. Pilates called his system "contrology," and control is a very important component of this exercise modality.

In the 1920s, Joe and his wife, Clara, immigrated to the United States and opened a studio in New York City. His work combines Eastern disciplines such as yoga and tai chi along with martial arts, boxing, and acrobatics. Contrology, now called Pilates, has mat exercises, exercises done on spring-based machines, and those that use small props such as rings and barrels.

In his book *Return to Life Through Contrology*, Pilates defined the benefits of his approach as more than just physical: " ... the acquirement of and enjoyment of physical well-being, mental, calm, and spiritual peace is priceless ... this unique trinity of a balanced body, mind, and spirit is the ideal to strive for ...."

BODY WISE

Pilates helps your back because it integrates proper skeletal alignment and strengthens core muscles (including the abdominals, shoulders, and hips).

Find a Good Teacher

You want someone who knows Pilates exercises and the human body. This is especially important for back pain prevention and rehab! Anyone can teach a cookie-cutter routine of exercises. Good teachers know the intent behind the exercises and can communicate them in a way that motivates and resonates with you. Good teachers also practice what they preach, have a sound understanding of body mechanics and anatomy, and tailor private sessions to meet a client's particular needs. They will challenge you while keeping you safe.

BODY WISE

"In 10 sessions you will feel the difference, in 20 you will see the difference, in 30 you will have a whole new body." —Joseph Pilates

Referrals from friends and other health-care professionals are always helpful. Like finding a good doctor, you want your Pilates instructor to be in sync with your personality and needs. Many Pilates studios offer introductory rates that enable you to try a few sessions and perhaps a few instructors before you commit to more sessions.

Training and Certifications

Like yoga, Pilates has evolved through time. Today, there are a variety of approaches, but core muscle development is fundamental to them all. Among the most well-known and respected trademarked brands are BASI, Balanced Body, Polestar Pilates, the Physical Mind Institute, Stott, and Romana's Pilates. Instructors can be certified through any of these trademarked brands or smaller studios that have their own training centers. Both are legitimate ways to learn.

What's most important is how many hours of training an instructor has received. The most comprehensive and credible programs require at least 300 hours of training, which includes anatomy, personal practice, observing other instructors working with clients, and practice-teaching of clients. The best programs also require that the students have themselves practiced Pilates and have had many hours of private instruction before they enter a Pilates training program.

When shopping for good Pilates instructors, ask about their hours of training, years of professional experience, areas of specialization (some do specialize in rehab), and continuing education. It takes about two years to become a well-trained, comprehensive Pilates instructor. Continuing education keeps instructors fresh and motivated in their work.

BODY WISE

The Pilates Method Alliance (PMA) is the international, not-for-profit, professional association dedicated to the teachings of Joseph H. and Clara Pilates. In addition to certification from local studios, an instructor might choose to also become PMA-certified. This national certification reflects that the instructor has been rigorously trained and has proven, in-depth knowledge of anatomy; Pilates equipment; and exercises. To sit for the exam, an instructor must have at least 450 hours of training.

Studios that are training centers may also be PMA-certified, showing their adherence to the high standards of the PMA.

Many instructors start their Pilates careers teaching mat classes. Certifications for teaching mat requires fewer hours than comprehensive training because there are no machines involved. The best mat certification programs have prerequisites such as personal Pilates experience and fitness teaching. These top programs typically require about 100 hours of training, which includes anatomy, observation, practice teaching, and demonstrated physical review.

As mentioned previously, an instructor can be mat- or equipment-certified. (Equipment certification is also called comprehensive certification.)

Mat vs. Machine

Pilates originally was principally a one-on-one training system. Today, most people are introduced to Pilates through mat classes. There are benefits to both, but, to truly understand the work and gain the benefits, you can't beat private sessions on the machines. The springs both support and challenge you. Most of all, with good instruction, you're taught how to work correctly. Just a few sessions will completely change your mat workout and bring better body awareness to all you do. If you can, we recommend you get a few private machine sessions. Here are just a few advantages to using Pilates machines:

- Spring-based machines assist and challenge deep core muscles. Instructor ensures proper alignment and technique.

- Machine assistance increases range of motion.

- The machine settings are customized to your needs, fitness, and goals.

DIY Resources

Whether you want to supplement your workouts or are curious to see what this Pilates thing is all about, there are some great recorded programs out there. In particular, look for DVDs from Stott Pilates and Balanced Body. Many libraries have exercise DVDs, so you can try before you buy. Likewise, YouTube has Pilates clips from various schools and instructors.

BODY WISE

Engaging your pelvic floor (the muscle you use to stop the flow of urine) helps you better contract and use your abdominal muscles.

Core Principles

The principles are the same regardless of whether you practice on a mat or machines. And even though there are some variations among styles of Pilates, they all focus on developing strength and flexibility by stabilizing core muscles. The main emphasis is quality of movement over quantity. Other unifying principles include:

- **Articulation:** Moving one vertebra at a time, mainly as you roll up or down in a movement.

- **Breath:** Full inhales and exhales help you connect with your core and energize and revitalize body, mind, and spirit.

- **Concentration:** The mind and body connect to improve focus and awareness. You have to think about what you're doing and feel how your muscles are working.

- **Control:** Movements are neither jerky nor fast.

- **Flow:** Exercises are fluid, not static or isolated. We move in space.

- **Precision:** Each exercise has unique benefits that are gained through focusing on the details.

- **Coordination:** In most exercises, one area of the body stabilizes while another part moves, requiring coordination and often balance.

- **Oppositions:** Using opposing forces develops strength, awareness, balance, and control.

BODY WISE

The general rule of thumb for breathing is to exhale on the exertion. In other words, inhale to prepare, exhale to move.

Core Moves

If you've been to physical therapy, some of the following exercises may be familiar to you, as Pilates moves are increasingly being incorporated into physical therapy. Some physical therapists are also Pilates instructors—a great combination for helping clients rehab and develop good exercise habits for life.

In Pilates, we always want the abs to draw in, never to protrude outward. That's true in every motion, forward, back, side to side, and twisting. The following Pilates exercises have been modified to a beginner level—but that doesn't mean they're easy! The point is to develop good form from the beginning.

Pelvic Tilts

These engage your deep core abdominal muscles, gain mobility in the hips, and gently massage your lower back.

BODY WISE

Abdominal muscles, or your abs, consist of four paired muscle groups. The deepest is the transversus abdominis, which hugs around your body like a corset and helps support your spine. When you pull in your belly to zip up tight jeans, these muscles are doing the work.

The internal obliques attach from your hips to your lower ribs. These muscles help you side bend and rotate and assist in forward bending. Above these muscles are the external obliques, which also enable side bending and rotation and assist in flexing the spine forward.

Rectus abdominis, better known as the six pack, is closer to the surface of your body. Even though most people don't have a sculpted six pack, the structure of three parallel muscles sets are still there. Its main function is to flex or pull your spine forward. When Pilates exercises are performed correctly, rectus abdominus helps to compress the belly down.

Begin on your back, knees bent, feet flat on the floor, arms down at your sides. Your hips should be in neutral alignment, meaning you're neither pressing your lower back into the floor nor are you arching your lower back.

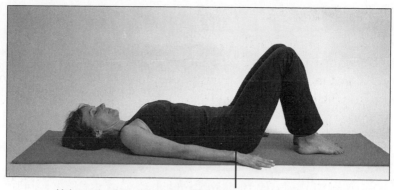

Using only ab muscles, draw your hips
(pelvis) toward you as belly pulls in.

Pelvic tilt.

On your exhale, gently pull your abdominal muscles in without gripping hard, then tip your hips toward you, curling your tailbone up through your legs. As you do this, your lower back touches the mat. This is a very small movement. The hips do not lift off the floor. Slowly return the hips to neutral (the natural curve in your lower back returns). Repeat several times.

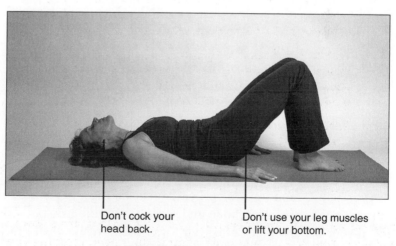

Don't cock your
head back.

Don't use your leg muscles
or lift your bottom.

Pelvic tilt common problems.

BODY WISE

Your deep core abdominal muscles (transversus abdominus) wrap around your body like a corset. If you place your hands around your center and cough, you'll feel these muscles and side ab muscles pull inward.

Engaging your pelvic floor (the muscle you use to stop the flow of urine) will help you connect with your deep core muscles.

Modified Roll Down

The purpose of this exercise is to strengthen your deep core abdominal muscles; your side abdominals assist.

Begin seated with your feet flat on the floor, hip-width apart, and not too close to your bottom. With your elbows out, sit tall on your sitting bones (knobby bones at your bottom).

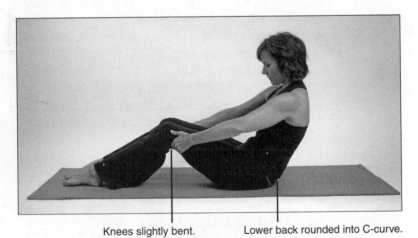

Knees slightly bent.   Lower back rounded into C-curve.

Modified roll down.

Pull your belly in and start to curl back (articulating one vertebra at a time as you draw your tailbone underneath you). Elbows stay wide. Look at your belly, roll down to your lower back, inhale, then slowly curl back up, returning to a tall position. Repeat five times.

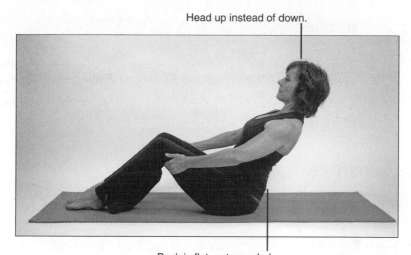

Head up instead of down.

Back is flat, not rounded.

Modified roll down common problems

Swan Prep

These strengthen your abdominal and back muscles and stretch the front of your body.

Begin face down, arms along sides with palms up, legs slightly apart in parallel position. Abdominals are pulled in, pubic bone slightly pressing down into mat.

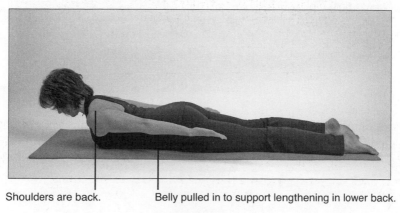

Shoulders are back.   Belly pulled in to support lengthening in lower back.

Swan prep.

Exhale while you straighten your arms, lift your upper back up, and lift your legs about an inch off the floor. Hips stay down. Be sure to pull your pelvic floor and belly in and slightly draw your tailbone through so you do not arch your lower back. Repeat five times.

If the movement bothers your lower back, don't lift your legs.

Head is back.

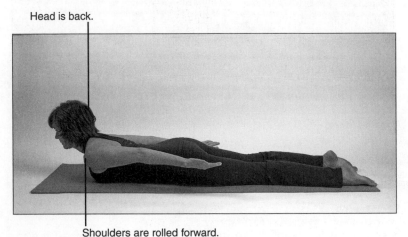

Shoulders are rolled forward.

Swan prep common problems.

Spine Twist

This strengthens side abdominals (obliques) and increases mobility in rotating the spine.

Begin seated with legs crossed and arms crossed in front of your chest and slightly lifted. Sit tall.

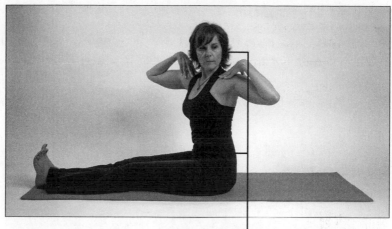

Keep spinal length as you twist; your head stays in the center of your body.

Spine twist.

Inhale to prepare, drawing your belly in as you exhale and twisting to your right. Return to center and repeat to other side. Do five repetitions to each side, alternating each time.

Shoulders roll forward instead of staying back.

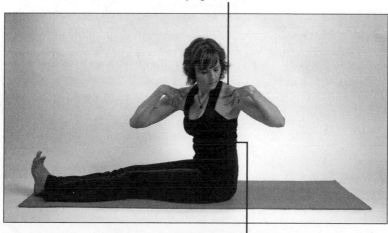

Spine shortens instead of lengthening while twisting.

Spine twist common problems.

Modified Mermaid

This strengthens side muscles (obliques) and creates flexibility in the spine while side bending.

Keep spinal length as you side bend.

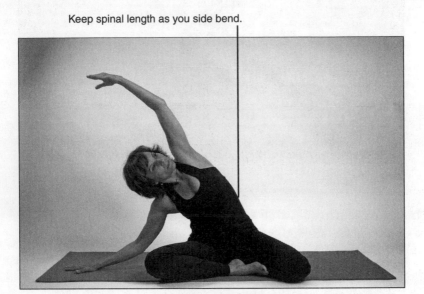

Modified mermaid.

Begin with your legs crossed and arms down at the sides. Keeping your legs relaxed, inhale to prepare, then exhale as you lift up and stretch to the side, using your arm to support your weight. The other arm lifts and reaches over your head. Slightly look up at the ceiling. Pause to inhale, then exhale to return to center. Do three repetitions. Recross your legs and repeat.

Shoulder lifts to the ear instead of staying relaxed down.

Spine moves forward instead of staying to the side.

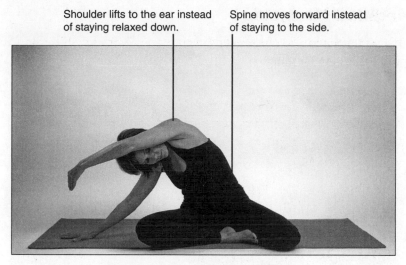

Modified mermaid common problems.

The Least You Need to Know

- Pilates is an excellent choice for building back and core muscles.
- Mat instructors should have at least 100 hours of training; comprehensive instructors (those that work with machines) should have at least 300 hours of training.
- Customized private sessions with a well-trained instructor will help you get further faster.

Ancient Wisdom of Yoga

In This Chapter

- The many benefits of yoga
- Criteria for choosing a teacher and a class
- Meditation and breath control techniques
- Back-specific exercises to help strengthen and stretch muscles

Originating in India, yoga is among the oldest mind-body exercises in the world. It works your core, enhances flexibility, and calms your mind. It's no wonder that it is so often recommended by health-care professionals. Yoga can be quite exciting and challenging. In this chapter, we'll share a few yoga exercises that will help you build core strength and flexibility as well as a few to help you relax.

When you have lower back problems, core stability muscles can begin to lose strength (a condition called muscle atrophy). Superficial muscles (those closer to the surface of the body) begin to take over and the deeper core muscles either shut off or the sequence of how muscles engage is incorrect. This sequencing is referred to as *muscle firing* in biomechanical lingo. To correct both misfiring patterns and muscle atrophy, you need to retrain muscles with mind-body awareness—a hallmark of yoga.

Movement and More

Yoga asks you to "multitask" in an interesting way. It requires proper focus, breath work, and concentrated precise poses appropriate to your body. Equally important in yoga (and in life), we need to let go of things we don't need, such as distracting thoughts or tensing muscles that aren't required for a movement.

Like any physical practice, yoga can make matters worse if it is not done carefully and wisely. Avoid any extreme positions such as back bends, extreme lateral bends, or head stands.

Types of Yoga

There are different styles of yoga. In general, those that are best for your back include hatha yoga and Iyengar yoga. Classes described as such will be more gentle and suitable to beginners. More rigorous styles of yoga include ashtanga and vinyasa, both of which flow more from position to position and require more strength and body awareness from the get go.

BODY WISE

Asanas (yoga poses) are held for several seconds or longer depending on the type of yoga you practice. The objective is to hold the position to become more aware of what you're feeling and adjust your body as needed. This is a key aspect of mind and body exercise.

Mats, Straps, Blocks

Most types of yoga use a mat, and some incorporate straps and blocks. These items, called props, can help you get into positions more easily. For example, if you are sitting and bending forward and can't reach your feet, a strap acts like an extension of your arms. Place the strap around your feet and you can gently pull yourself forward.

Find a Good Teacher

It's easy to feel intimidated by yoga when you see pictures of people bending themselves into pretzel shapes. This is not the average person's goal. The goal is to move at your own pace and place your body in a position that is right for you. A good instructor will never show off or create a competition to see which students can be more flexible. Rather, a good instructor is gentle, inviting, and encouraging to all students.

Training and Certifications

Certification is a rather new concept in the world of yoga. The tradition was that aspiring teachers trained with those whom they admired. Most practiced for years before teaching others. The training programs generally included understanding of anatomy as well as proficiency in personal practice and teaching others. Serious practitioner/teachers make the trek to India to study with masters there. Teachers who are truly into yoga make the practice an integral part of their lives.

THE BACK AND BEYOND

The exercises in yoga are only one part of a system of living developed in India thousands of years ago. The system includes training the mind, body, and spirit. Relaxation, diet, and meditation as well as daily exercise are included within yoga. It's not a religion; rather, it's a philosophy for living practiced by people of many religions.

When yoga became more popular and health clubs began offering classes, it became necessary to ensure that those who said they were yoga teachers were truly qualified. Many yoga-certification programs require that prospective teachers have at least a couple of years of practice under their belts before they begin training.

Look for teachers who have at least 200 hours of training and participate in continuing education. Ask them about their experience with back pain. They may or may not be a part of the national certifying body, *Yoga Alliance*. Older yoga teachers may have many more years' experience than ones who just began their careers and are certified through the Alliance. Your best bet is to take a class, do what feels good to you, and see whether you like the teaching style.

DEFINITIONS

Yoga Alliance is a nonprofit organization that established a national **Yoga Teachers' Registry** to recognize and promote teachers with training that meets minimum training standards (200 or 500 hours). The Yoga Alliance also maintains a school registry of those programs that meet its strict standards.

Pranayama Breath of Life

Breathing exercises, or pranayama, are an important part of yoga as they link the body with the mind. There are many different breathing practices; all help create mental clarity and emotional serenity. Find a comfortable place to sit where you won't be disturbed for at least five minutes.

Controlled Breathing

In this exercise, you are seeking to become aware of your breath by controlling the length of your inhalations and exhalations. In both cases, you are breathing through your nose. The practice itself is quite simple:

1. Breathe in slowly for a count of six (allow your belly to expand but don't push it out).

2. Hold for three counts.

3. Exhale slowly for a count of six (push all the air out using your abdominals).

4. Hold for three counts. Repeat the sequence several times.

As you build your lung capacity, you will be able to extend the inhales and exhales to longer counts. This practice is an ideal and easy way to reduce stress, prepare yourself for meetings, and help yourself fall asleep more easily.

Alternate Nostril Breathing

In this breathing exercise, the exhalation is twice the length of the inhalation. The purpose is to empty the lungs with the belief that you are also draining waste out of the body as well.

1. Using your right thumb, close the right nostril. Exhale out of the left nostril, then inhale deeply through it for a count of four.

2. Close the left nostril with your right ring or little finger and hold for eight counts.

3. Release the right nostril and exhale to an eight count.

4. With the left nostril now closed, inhale to a four count.

5. Close both nostrils and hold for eight counts.

6. Release the left nostril and exhale to an eight count.

The preceding is considered one cycle. It takes a bit of coordination to get the alternate breathing method down, but like most things in life, with practice it will become easier. Try to complete at least five cycles.

The Power of Meditation

Yoga is of course renowned for its meditation practices. As with the breathing exercises, there are many different ways to meditate. You may have heard meditation referred to as emptying your mind of thoughts. It's nearly impossible (even for long-time meditators) to sustain a mind clear of thought for a long time. We are born thinkers. The objective is to slow down the runaway train of thoughts and also to learn not to let our thoughts continuously carry us away from the present moment. It is a challenge to stay truly in the present. Most of the time, we are thinking about something in the past or ruminating about the future.

Think of a meditation practice as making deposits into a bank. For the greatest return, try to practice a few minutes daily. In the long run, the compounded benefits will enrich your life.

Mindfulness Meditation

Ideally, you want a quiet place where you will not be disturbed. In this practice, you simply want to become aware of your thoughts. Notice them but try not to let them carry you away. Some thoughts, such as, "What should I have for dinner?" are small distractions. Others can lead to full-fledged fantasy conversations. Either way, you want to notice them and gently nudge your mind back to the moment.

Using your senses to bring you back to the moment can be helpful. Notice the sounds that are around you—those that are near, those that are farther away. This can bring you back to the present moment.

THE BACK AND BEYOND

Studies have shown that regular meditation can reduce depression, which makes chronic pain worse. The practice helps you stay present and less likely to anticipate negative future events.

Focused Meditation

Much like breathing exercises, in focused meditation, the practitioner focuses on something. That something could be the breath—noticing minute details of how it feels. For example, feel the air tickle through the nostrils; take note of how the air expands the belly and lungs. The focus could also be sounds such as repeating a prayer or a simple phrase such as, "I breathe in energy, I exhale and release frustration." You could also focus visually, such as on a candle, watching the colors and flame flicker and shift.

Meditation in Action

You can practice meditation throughout your day even if you can't break away to solitude. It's a matter of noticing and using common events to remind you to stay present. For example, when you are driving, you can use red lights or stop signs as metaphors for you to take a moment to check in with your thoughts. Likewise, when the phone rings, let it bring you back to the present. Don't anticipate what you will and won't say. Stay alert in the present moment and let the conversation unfold calmly.

Strike a Pose with Asanas

Mind-body yoga exercises are an excellent way to strengthen your core and subsequently reduce common aches and pains. No two people's poses will ever be alike because no two bodies are exactly alike. Approach these with gentleness and avoid pushing your body into extremes of any position.

As with any exercise and back pain or rehab, if you are unsure whether a position is right for you, consult your health-care practitioner.

Bridging

This strengthens core and back muscles and gently massages your spine.

Begin on your back, knees bent, feet flat on the floor, arms down at your sides. A block between your knees is useful but not essential. The block will help you engage your inner thighs.

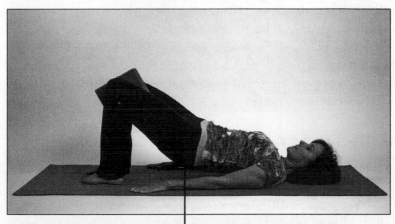

Draw your hips forward and slowly lift your hips up toward the ceiling.

Bridging.

On your exhale, gently pull your abdominal muscles in, curl your tailbone up through your legs, and lift your hips up toward the ceiling. Stop when you reach your shoulder blades. Hold to inhale, then slowly lower your spine down vertebra by vertebra, keeping the weight distribution even on both sides of your back. Repeat several times.

> **WATCH YOUR BACK**
>
> Don't let your hips sag down and create stress in the lower back.

Seated Spine Twist

This works the rotator muscles and creates more flexibility in the spine.

Begin seated with one leg bent, the other straight.

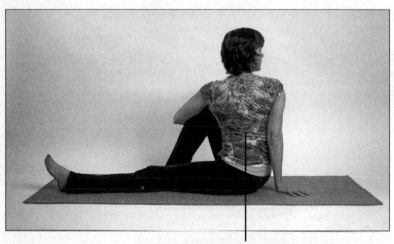

Rotate with a lengthened spine turning to look over the shoulder in the direction of your twist.

Seated spine twist.

With the right leg bent, wrap your left arm around your knee, rotate, and place your right arm behind you with your palm on the floor. Hold to inhale, and as you exhale, slowly return to center. Repeat several times to each side.

Cat/Cow

This works the abdominal muscles and creates flexibility in the spine. Done in sequence, these poses work the spine in opposite directions—gentle forward bends and back bends.

Begin on your hands and knees with your hands in line with your shoulders and knees in line with your hips; your spine remains neutral (neither extended nor flexed).

In cat, the spine is flexed (rounded).

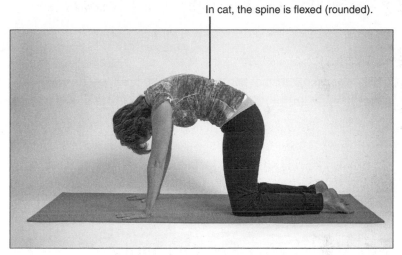

Cat.

In cow, the spine is gently extended (arched).

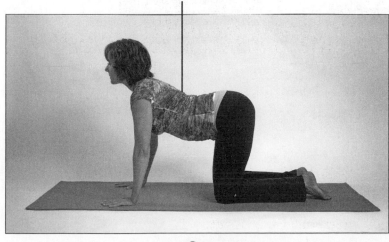

Cow.

Inhale to prepare; as you exhale, pull your tailbone under as you round your spine looking down and through your legs. Pause. Inhale as you slowly move the spine into an arched position, drawing your shoulders back and looking up toward the ceiling. Return to neutral. Repeat several times.

WATCH YOUR BACK

In cow, be careful not to just drop into an arched lower back. It is a gentle arch held securely in place with your abdominal muscles.

Pigeon

This is a wonderful stretch for the legs and helps loosen the hip joints. It is especially helpful for counterbalancing the effects of sitting.

Begin on your hands and knees. Place your right knee toward your right hand, extend your left leg back.

Bring your elbows to the floor and feel the stretch in your right hip. To increase the stretch, you can fold your body forward and place your head on the floor. Hold for several seconds, then move to the opposite side.

Hips are square; gaze is forward and down.

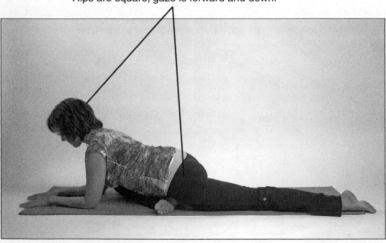

Pigeon.

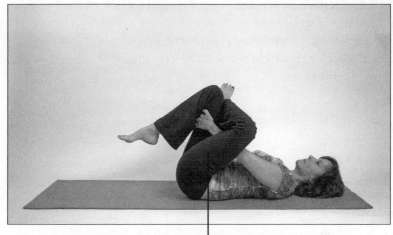

To stretch the same muscle group, you can also lie on your back, cross one ankle over your knee, and gently pull your legs toward you.

Pigeon 2.

Happy Baby Pose

This stretches hip flexor muscles, releasing their pull on your back.

Begin on your back, both legs up and knees angled narrow to your body. Reach to the outside of your feet and firmly pull the feet down toward the floor. Your knees will not reach the floor. Hold the position for several seconds. Release and experience the opening in your hips. Most people report that their legs feel longer after this exercise.

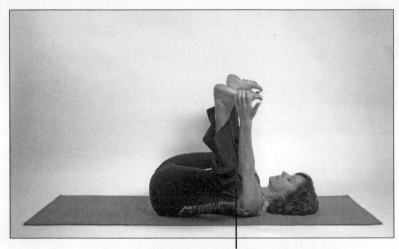

Be sure to angle your legs just to the outside of
your body so you can pull the legs down.

Happy baby pose.

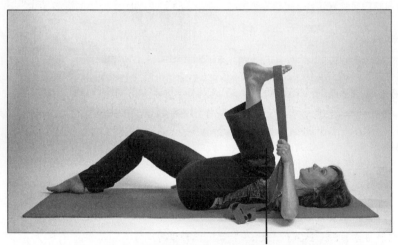

This pose can also be done with one leg at a time,
using the strap to help you pull the leg down.

Happy baby pose, single-leg version.

Hamstring Stretch

This stretches the hamstrings, the muscles on the back of your legs. These can get tight from sitting and also from activities such as running.

Begin on your back, one leg up with a strap around the foot.

Gently draw the leg toward your head, trying to keep the knee as straight as possible. The opposite leg can be bent or straight, depending on your flexibility. Hold for several seconds on each side.

Reaching your heel up toward the ceiling intensifies the stretch.

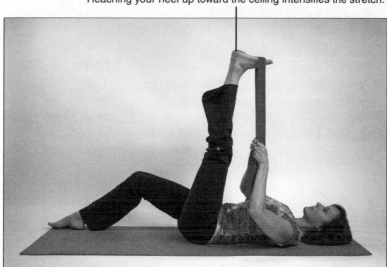

Hamstring stretch.

The Least You Need to Know

- Yoga can help back problems by stretching and strengthening muscles.
- Not all styles of yoga are appropriate for those rehabbing from back injury or surgery, or just getting started in yoga.
- Yogic breathing and meditation techniques reduce stress and can calm stress-related back problems.

Health Clubs and Home Workouts

In This Chapter

- Combining core and functional training
- Personal trainer certifications and specialties
- Exercise essentials
- Challenging your balance, and conditioning and stretching your muscles

There's nothing like an expert fitness assessment, but we all share some common daily-life movements. We sit. We stand. We walk. We mow the lawn. We run to catch the bus, hoping not to spill our coffee along the way. For this, we need the core and more. In this chapter, we offer you some exercise ideas that support your core and everyday movements.

Find a Good Personal Trainer

For some time now, core and *functional training* have been all the rage in the world of fitness. These approaches are worth their weight in buzz because they help people function better in daily life. Core training and functional training are two sides of the same coin. Both focus on developing muscles to support daily activities, reducing the chances of injuring or reinjuring your back.

> **DEFINITIONS**
>
> **Functional training** refers to exercises that support what you do every day, such as standing, picking up children, or climbing up stairs. Well-designed programs build strength and flexibility that enhance natural movements and coordination between muscles and the nervous system.

Each person is a unique musculoskeletal package with specific daily activities. Personal trainers are experts who specialize in core and functional training and carefully assess a client's daily activities to create a custom exercise routine.

Training and Certifications

Personal trainer certification is the norm in health clubs, gyms, and community centers such as the YMCA. Be aware, however, that one can become a certified personal trainer in a relatively short period of time (such as a long weekend). Among the better training/certifying agencies are the American Council on Exercise (ACE), the National Academy of Sports Medicine (NASM), and the American College of Sports Medicine (ACSM). They generally have more stringent programs and testing. All require continuing education to stay certified.

> **BODY WISE**
>
> Many trainers have college degrees in exercise science, where they study such subjects as anatomy, physiology, and kinesiology (human movement).

Experienced trainers tend to specialize in certain populations such as elderly, athletes, or boomers and/or in types of exercise such as prenatal or post rehab (picking up where physical therapists leave off). Talk with prospective trainers about their education, specialization, and experience. Many have reduced-price introductory offers. It's best to try a session or two before committing to longer packages. It might go without saying, but we'll say it anyway: the ideal personal trainer should "walk the walk." They should move well and be fit and healthy. This doesn't mean model thin or bulging with massive muscles. In fact, overly trained muscles aren't functional—they're too tight. You can easily see it when muscle-bound people try to do simple things such as bending down; overly tight muscles restrict motions.

Power Up with Resistance Training

There are many ways to create resistance to condition your muscles: with your own body such as with push-ups, through weight-training with bar bells, and by using flexible bands. All will increase your strength.

BODY WISE

When performing resistance exercises, you want to exhale on the exertion. That means exhaling on the hardest part of the exercise. For example, when doing bicep curls, you inhale to prepare, then exhale when you lift the weight up.

There is a difference between free weights and machines. Free weights require more control. You have to balance and support the weight as you move it. Machines, on the other hand, help support the movement, which can be an advantage when beginning a weight training program.

WATCH YOUR BACK

To get the most from your exercise routine, good form is essential. Slowly lifting and releasing, supporting the spine by using abdominals, and using weights that you can control will go a long way toward keeping your back safe while conditioning your muscles. Proper form not only builds better muscles, but does so with less chance of injury.

How much should you lift and how often? In general, you'll want to complete three sets of a given exercise. Each set should consist of 8 to 10 repetitions. By the end of the last set, your targeted muscles should feel fatigued. Work each muscle group twice a week. For example, on Mondays and Wednesdays, work the lower body; on Tuesdays and Thursdays, work the upper body.

Muscle Conditioning with Resistance Bands

Flexible bands have an advantage in that they're light and portable and come in various resistances. You can work legs, arms, and abdominal muscles with these bands. You can also easily use them for a quick pick-me-up at the office or on the road. As we've said before, short bursts of exercise throughout the day do make a difference. Here are three quick and easy ways to use these bands.

Hold the flex band loosely. Keep your wrists straight. Don't wrap the band around your hand. To increase resistance, grab closer to the middle. To decrease resistance, hold closer to the ends. Stand up straight and draw your abdominals in. The basic breathing pattern for all exercises is inhale to prepare and exhale to lift.

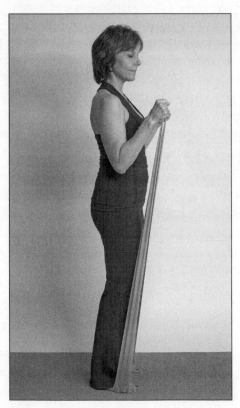

Biceps curls and core power.

Stand on the middle of the band with one end in each hand. Standing tall, lift the band up slowly, then slowly lower it down. Do 10 reps. Pause and repeat twice.

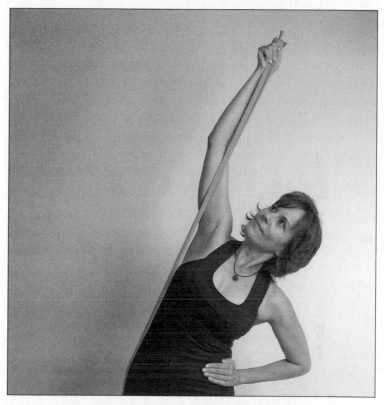

Side stretch and strength.

Step on one end of the band with your right heel. Grasp the other end of the band with your right hand. The band should be taut as you lift it straight up, shoulder down (not up toward your ears). Side bend slowly to the left and slowly return to center. Exhale as you bend to the side. Do five reps. Repeat to other side.

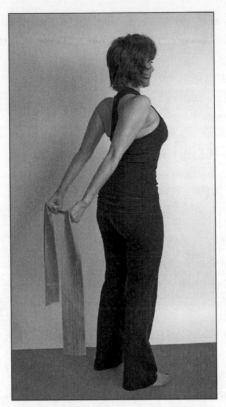

Upper back opener and tricep strengthener.

Hold the band behind your back, palms facing away from you, hands close together. Roll your shoulders back. With your arms straight, pull the band down and apart while slightly arching the upper back. Do five reps. Pause and repeat. This exercise is perfect for relieving stress from computer work!

Get Balanced

Focusing on balance-building exercises is especially important as we age. We need balance for many daily activities. If you live in a cold climate with ice and snow, good balance will help prevent you from slipping. And if you do fall, a strong core will help minimize injury.

There are many fun ways to challenge your balance. As with muscle conditioning, you can simply use your own body (stand on one leg, for example) or you try one of the many inexpensive gadgets on the market or at your gym. They include:

- Wobble boards

- Rotating disks

- Rocker-bottom walking shoes

Importance of Low-Impact Aerobics

In addition to conditioning muscles and improving your balance, activities that increase your heart rate also help keep your back in tip-top shape. How? To stay in good condition, your spine and inter-vertebral discs need good blood flow. Aerobic activity increases blood flow throughout your body. The increased heart rate helps spread the natural endorphins your body releases in response to exercise.

To get the most bang from your aerobic exercise buck, aim for at least 3 weekly sessions of 30 minutes. How do you know whether you're at the right heart rate? In general if you can talk but can't sing, you're good. Here are some low-impact aerobic choices:

- Bicycle

- Swim

- Power walk

- Elliptical machine

- Nonimpact dance

BODY WISE

Supporting your sport of choice with exercises that stretch and strengthen often-used muscles is a smart way to reduce injury and better your per-formance. For example, golfers would do well to add exercises that improve the flexibility and strength of spinal rotator muscles; dancers need flexible and strong legs, feet, and abdominal muscles; and swim-mers require strong and flexible shoulders.

Get on the Ball

With these large, inflatable balls, you can get some aerobic exercise as well as core conditioning. To increase your heart rate, just bounce on the ball. It's fun. Be sure to keep your spine supported by engaging your abdominal muscles. Always be in control of your bounce. You are bouncing the ball, the ball is not bouncing you! While you are bouncing, you also have to balance (if you weren't balancing, you'd fall off). Here are some other back-benefiting ways to use an inflatable ball.

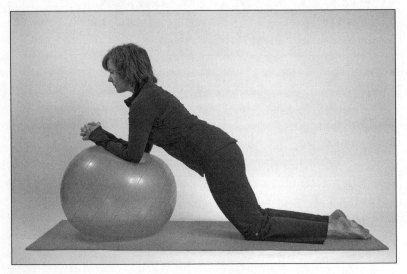

Kneeling core challenge.

Kneel in front of the ball and place your elbows on it. Gently press down, keeping your shoulders down and away from your ears. Slightly pull your tailbone under and lean forward into the ball without letting your torso touch the ball. Don't arch your back! This exercise works all your abdominal muscles and also your shoulders.

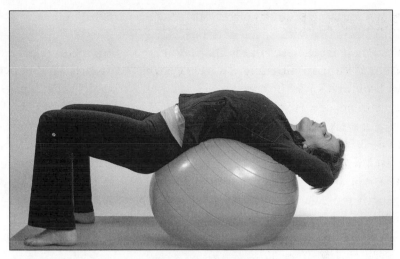

Supported back bend.

Lay backward on the ball with your feet parallel and hip-width apart. Support your head with your hands; allow your upper back to arch back a little. The farther back you go, the deeper the stretch. This helps open your chest and shoulders, which often get tight from sitting.

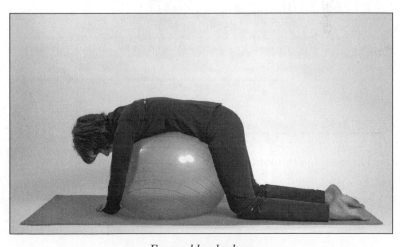

Forward bend release.

From a kneeling position, place your body over the ball, allowing your spine to take the shape of the ball. This is a wonderful way to relax and open the back of the spine. You are flexing the back, which is a good thing to do unless you have a herniated disc that is causing you problems.

Stretch It Out with a Foam Roller

As we mentioned in Chapter 5, the foam roller is a wonderful device to have on hand. You can do many exercises with it. Some build strength and balance; others increase flexibility. Here are two feels-so-good positions to try.

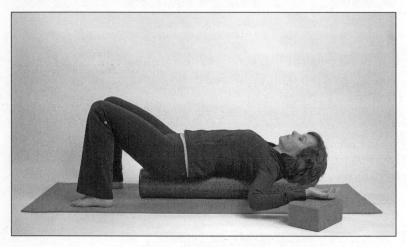

Chest and shoulder opener.

Lie down on the roller with your arms in the goal-post position. To relax most effectively, you want your hands to touch the floor. If your chest and shoulders are too tight to reach the floor, you can place pillows under your hands. Remain in the position for a minute or more. Breathe slowly and calmly. This position releases muscles that tighten from sitting.

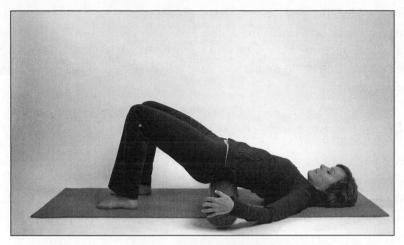

Lower back and hip release.

Position the roller underneath your sacrum, the triangular-shaped bone at the bottom of your spine. There are a lot of nerve endings at this point, so it may be a little tender, in a hurts-so-good kind of way. It should not be painful, however. You can simply hold the position shown here. For a greater hip stretch, draw one leg in toward you and the other one straight out. Hold the position for about a minute, then switch legs. The position stretches tight hip muscles, often a cause of lower back pain.

The Least You Need to Know

- To strengthen muscles, you can use weights, resistance bands, large inflatable balls, and/or other devices.
- The ideal fitness approach for back care includes aerobics, muscle conditioning, balance work, and stretching.
- To avoid injury, good form is essential in all exercises.

Ergonomics: Aligned in Life

In This Chapter

- Solutions for daily back pain culprits
- Why ergonomics matter and how to make simple adjustments at home, work, and play
- Getting a good night's sleep

When it comes to back pain, the little things can often snowball into larger problems: a forward head position at the computer, slouching while standing, sleeping on a saggy mattress.

In this chapter, we encourage you to take a closer look at your body in daily life. You'll likely discover some adjustments you can make to help reduce back pain and reinjury by keeping your body in better alignment. It's not hard to do; you just have to be aware of what you are doing, how you are doing it, and what adjustments you need to make.

Three Keys

A simple approach to proper alignment is to think about maintaining your natural spinal curves during any task or sedentary position. When your spine is aligned, you don't need much muscle strength to maintain it. Conversely, when you are sitting with poor posture, the muscles supporting you are chronically contracting. That exhausts your body and can lead to muscle spasms.

We're going to talk about three key concepts:

- **Posture:** How you hold yourself in static positions such as sitting or standing

- **Body mechanics:** The alignment of your body when you move

- **Ergonomics:** Modifying an environment to align with your body

All three help evenly distribute your weight, which keeps your spine happily aligned.

At Work

Every job has its unique physical challenges. Those that involve prolonged sitting can be as hard on the back as those that require lifting. Fortunately, there are some simple solutions. Of course, life and jobs don't line up perfectly into the following categories, but we think you'll gain a good perspective on how best to move your body for the variety of positions that your job may require.

Computer and Desk Jobs

Both posture and ergonomics come into play here. If you constantly lean in toward the monitor because you can't see well, both your neck and back will be unhappy. The following illustration outlines how to make your work space back-friendly.

Every decade, a new kind of chair makes the rounds for back pain. In the 1980s, the fad was those kneeling chairs; in the 1990s, exercise balls were big. Now the mesh support chair is popular. Any of these are good options, but sitting on the exercise ball is probably the best for overall core strengthening. Still, don't think you can or should be sitting on the ball all day, that would probably be fatiguing. Instead, alternate between the ball and a conventional chair.

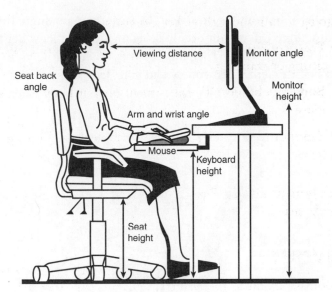

Working at the computer.

Prolonged Sitting

Cab drivers, truckers, and airline pilots all sit for long periods, which wreaks havoc on the back. If your seat doesn't provide lower back support, lumbar support cushions are helpful (you can use them on office chairs, too).

WATCH YOUR BACK

Auto collisions can lead to whiplash. To reduce the incidence, ensure that your headrest is just a couple of inches behind your head when you're seated in your regular driving position. The height of the rest should align with the top of your head.

Other ways to avoid risk of back strain while driving include sitting upright, placing both hands on the wheel, and keeping the back pockets empty. Sitting on a wallet stuffed to the brim will misalign your hip position. Not a happy place to be! Shifting your weight and using the cruise control option are also helpful in reducing excess pressure on the spine.

If you have tilt options for your seat, be sure that you angle the seat to distribute the weight evenly on your hips and legs. Set the distance to your pedals so that you can press them while your knee remains slightly bent when you extend your leg.

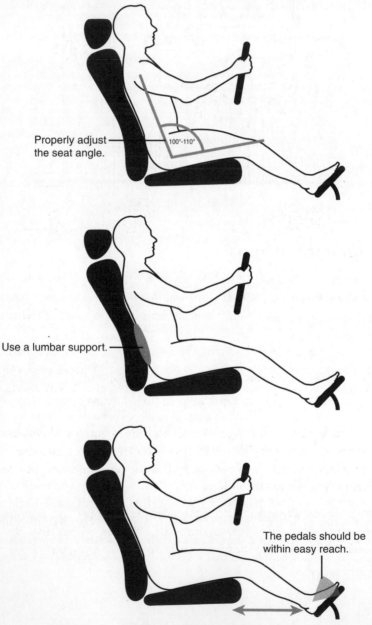

Properly adjust the seat angle.

100°-110°

Use a lumbar support.

The pedals should be within easy reach.

Vehicle seat adjustments.

Jobs That Require Lifting

To reduce risk of injury when lifting, you want to bend your knees (not your back), hold the object close to your body, and avoid lifting any higher than shoulder level. This is as true on the job as it is at home. You should lift a child or a bag of groceries the same way.

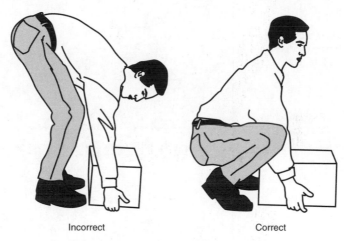

Incorrect   Correct

Proper lifting technique.

Prolonged Standing

Teachers, restaurant staff, factory workers, and many health-care professionals work on their feet all day. Many of them (a surgeon, for example) also have to bend forward and look down. When we stand, we want to keep the spine aligned as much as possible.

Avoid slouching the shoulders when bending forward and also avoid the opposite. Thrusting the chest forward can hyperextend the lower back and cause strain. Try using a foot stool and alternate your feet to shift weight between the hips.

Large-breasted women should wear a properly supportive brassiere. Some women undergo breast reduction surgeries, which may be covered by insurance if that is believed to be a component of their back pain.

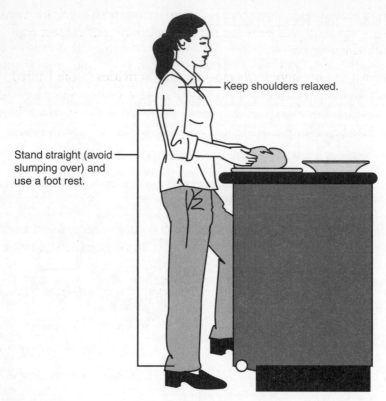

Keep shoulders relaxed.

Stand straight (avoid slumping over) and use a foot rest.

Standing technique.

At Play

The days of swinging from the monkey bars may (or may not) be long gone for you, but you probably do enjoy many leisure activities. Whether you watch sports or participate in activities, keep the following tips in mind.

Moving It

Sports, like jobs, all have their unique demands. We talked a bit in previous chapters about the importance of training your muscles to support your favorite activities. You also need to pay attention to your posture and biomechanics while doing these activities, too.

Tips from pros are always useful. A few lessons with a golf or tennis pro, for example, will help you get your game on and correct common posture problems, too.

Believe it or not, among the most popular activities in the United States is power walking, and it's a great, back-friendly exercise choice. But again, it's one of those innocent-looking activities in which back pain may be lurking. Here are a few walking tips to keep in mind:

- Keep your body upright (don't lean forward).

- Align your head atop of your shoulders, eyes looking forward (not down). Keep your neck relaxed.

- Keep your elbows bent (no more than 90 degrees) and hands relaxed. Don't excessively swing your arms; instead, allow a natural swing to occur.

Your heels should reach the ground first and your foot should simply roll through the stride.

BODY WISE

Proper fitting shoes are a must for any sport. Here's what you need to know to get the best fit.

- Stand up while your feet are measured, and buy shoes near the end of the day, when feet are likely to be a bit larger.

- Make sure that your shoes aren't so tight that they pinch your toes, but they shouldn't be so big that they slide around on your feet.

- Don't purchase shoes that feel too tight, expecting them to "stretch" to fit.

- Bend the shoe; it should "break" under the big toe area, not the middle of the shoe.

In the Bleachers

Can simply watching a sporting event wreck your back? Yes, if you're lying about on sagging cushions or in bleacher seats with no back rests. Invest in a new couch or repair those cushions (it's cheaper and less painful than trying to fix your back). And next time you're at a sporting event, take a chair with a built-in back rest. They're inexpensive, portable, and commonly available online. Simply search for bleacher seats with back rests.

At Home

Every day you wake up, wash your face, brush your teeth, have breakfast (we hope), and continue your day. Come evening, it's relaxation time, for most people on the couch or in front of a computer. When it comes to lights out, falling asleep may be a challenge if you have back pain. And you'll want to be sure that your sleep position doesn't make you wake up grouchy with pain.

> **WATCH YOUR BACK**
>
> Stress can cause and worsen back pain and prevent you from getting a good night's sleep. Worry about financial issues, anxiety over important meetings and presentations, or anger at your spouse or kids creates tension in the body. Calm your emotional reactions with meditation or breathing techniques (see Chapter 16) and you'll fall asleep more easily.

Sleeping and Waking

We've all seen those mattress commercials promising a good night's sleep. We're not going to advocate any particular brand, but we are going to agree that a good mattress that supports your spine's natural curves is best for your back.

If you have trouble falling asleep, limit or eliminate caffeine and alcohol. Your room should be dark and quiet. As far as your best back-friendly sleep positions, here are some tips. If you sleep on your side, place a pillow between your knees to keep your hips in a neutral position. If you're most comfortable on your back, a pillow under your knees relieves pressure on your lower back by gently flexing your hips. Avoid sleeping on your stomach, as it can hyperextend your back and neck.

When you wake, roll over to the side of your bed, boost your self up with your arm as you release your legs over the edge. Don't just pop up straight out of bed. If you've ever watched a cat or dog, they leisurely stretch a bit then get up. We'd be wise to do the same.

Intimacy

If your back pain has you concerned about your love life, you're not alone. But your relationship does not have to suffer. You may have to put it off for a little while, and when you return to physical love, you may have to take it easy and try some new positions.

But why not make the return a good excuse to experiment playfully with new positions? Talk about fun! This is your chance to truly make lemonade from lemons. Of course, get your doctor's approval regarding when and how to return, especially if you're recovering from back surgery. Get your pillows ready! The next chapter details back-friendly ways to maintain your intimate life.

Washing Up

Slouching is every back's enemy, so check yourself when you're at the sink. When washing your face, don't bend your back; bend your knees. When you shave or apply makeup, bring the mirror to you instead of leaning into it. Wall-mounted magnifying mirrors that swivel are perfect for this. If you have to bend over the sink, support part of your weight with one outstretched arm. Stand close to the sink as well so you don't have to lean into it. Most kitchen and bathroom cabinets have a kickboard cutout designed to let you stand closer. Use it!

Watching TV

There's nothing like being a couch potato after a long, hard day. But as we've already mentioned, you want to keep your back happy when watching your favorite shows. That means supportive cushions. If you're sitting, be sure your lower back is supported with a lumbar roll or pillow and keep your feet flat on the floor. If you want to kick your feet up, they should not go higher than your hips. A little elevation is good, but you can get too much of a good thing and strain your back needlessly.

And if you're looking for a way to sneak more exercise into your day (we're all for that), use the time during commercials to get active instead of getting another handful of potato chips. You can stretch or do sit-up or push-up competitions with others in the room. Of course, be sure you're using proper form in any exercise you do.

The Least You Need to Know

- How you walk, sit, stand, and sleep can create or reduce back pain.
- You can adjust your work and home environments to better fit your body.
- Incorporate back-friendly items into your life, such as lumbar support rolls, magnifying swivel mirrors, and supportive mattresses.

It Takes Two: Sex and Pregnancy

In This Chapter

- How back pain can improve intimacy
- Personality profiles and communication styles
- Creating romance and desire
- Back-friendly sex positions

Anger, frustration, depression. These are hardly the ingredients for a good sex life. But you can expect these emotions with back pain, especially if it's chronic. No wonder partners often find themselves irritated with the situation and with one another.

But what if we were to tell you that back pain can actually lead to *better* sex and intimacy? Don't close the book. In fact, keep this chapter earmarked and on your night table. Sex is important to your relationship and your health. Whether you have the back issue or your partner does, one of the easiest ways to get started on your journey back to sexual intimacy is for *both* of you to read this chapter.

Reality Check

Pain can affect a man's sexual performance. Sometimes, it's psychological; other times, it is truly physical. When it's psychological, a man may feel that he is not the strong, healthy man his lover needs him to be and thus he feels emasculated in the bedroom. Other times, chronic pain can physically impair sexual readiness. It is difficult for a man to get or maintain an erection when his body is focused on severe pain. He has to be and feel relaxed to enjoy the experience. Pain medications can also markedly affect a man's performance.

> **THE BACK AND BEYOND**
>
> Men who undergo back surgery from an anterior approach (through the abdomen) are at risk for a condition called retrograde ejaculation. The nerves that send semen out of the penis during an orgasm are very sensitive. The approach for surgery can affect those nerves and sometimes the ejaculation goes into the bladder instead of exiting the penis. Although the orgasm still occurs, it is very difficult for such men to father a child. For other men, the lack of a visible release is also quite disheartening.

The same is true for women, but in a different light. It's hard for a woman with back pain to prance around in heels and a slinky nightgown when she really wants to sit back in sweats and slippers. For a woman with back pain, the physical act of intercourse can exacerbate the pain and make the entire experience less than desirable. To form proper lubrication and be at ease, women, like men, need to be relaxed and not focused on their pain.

That's why it's so important you talk about these issues. Don't leave your partner in the dark. He or she may misinterpret your avoidance of sex as a lack of desire for him or her.

> **WATCH YOUR BACK**
>
> Get your doctor's approval before returning to sex. Discuss positions that would be best and those that you should avoid. It's okay. Doctor's get such questions all the time. If your doctor doesn't mention the topic, initiate the conversation.

We Need to Talk

These words can bring such anxiety in a relationship. But as another cliché says, communication is the key to a good and lasting relationship. The more openly two people can communicate, the better. That, of course, is easier said than done. How we communicate with one another can lead to successful understanding or drive us further into frustration. One way to get to know yourself and your partner better is through the work of Swiss psychiatrist Carl Jung.

When he was a young doctor, Jung collaborated with famed psychiatrist Sigmund Freud (famous for his theory that sex is a primary motivator in life). The duo's paths diverged when Jung delved deeper into defining and categorizing the psyche, which basically means the life force that drives behaviors, thoughts, and reactions. If you've ever taken a Myers-Briggs Type Indicator test (some jobs require it), much of it was created using Jung's ideas.

> **BODY WISE**
>
> Myers-Briggs Type Indicator tests are readily available online. It would be revealing and instructive to you and your relationship if you both took the test and shared the results. It's an insightful and interesting exercise.

First, Know Yourself

What does all this have to do with back pain and communication? The better you know yourself and your partner, the better you can talk to one another. This section presents a broad summary of Jung's four functions, which are present in all of us. The functions are how we approach the world. The difference is which function do we lead with and which lies deeper in our unconscious.

The Jungian typological functions are ranked in each individual. The first function is our primary driver. We lead with that function. The second is less so but still quite a strong working function. The latter two reside in our unconscious, making the third and fourth functions less developed in our personalities.

Jung theorized that as we get to middle age, a shift occurs as the psyche strives toward wholeness. For example, those who have thinking as their first function and feeling as their unconscious fourth function will find that as they get older, they will start to lead more from their hearts and less from their minds.

THE BACK AND BEYOND

Jung further classifies personality as introverted and extroverted, terms which he coined. In the Jungian definition, an extrovert is a person who is more outwardly oriented and finds meaning in the surrounding world. This person has a greater need to be around people; it's a motivating force. The introvert is more reclusive and finds greater meaning within himself or herself.

The following subsections present the four functions as they would manifest in the primary position. Understanding a person's basic orientation to the world can lead to more efficient, effective communication.

Thinking

Those whose primary function is thinking are analytical and conceptual and tend to be well organized. They can sometimes seem detached and unemotional. That's because for many thinkers, feelings are the most challenging function. In fact, emotions can be quite overwhelming for thinkers.

Therefore, when communicating with people whose primary function is as a thinker, it's best to approach them with language that is more logical than emotional. "If we set time aside to discuss sex, we can improve it."

Feeling

Those who primarily experience life through their feelings approach the world from the opposite way that thinkers do. They are empathetic and lead with their hearts rather than their heads.

Approach the sex conversation from the perspective of feelings. For example, "If we take some time to talk about sex, we can improve our intimacy and feel closer to one another."

Sensate

People who lead with the sensate function live in the present moment. They are focused on the now: their hunger, their thirst, or their desire for sex, now. Therefore, a good time to talk about sex may be when the person desires it. But be ready to have your needs clearly defined in a physical sense. If you are the one with the back pain, have those pillows nearby and the positions to try at the ready (see the "Positioned for Fun" section later in this chapter).

> **BODY WISE**
>
> A thinker is opposite from a feeler; a sensate is opposite from an intuitive. Good to know, because opposites often attract!

Intuition

People who lead with intuition are quick to learn new things and are great at multitasking (unlike the sensate, who is best doing one thing at a time). They are often "not in their bodies"; rather, they tend to daydream and jump around from thought to thought. They like the new. They lead by gut reaction. An approach to the talk might be something like, "Let's talk about some creative new ways to approach our sex life."

Candid and Successful Conversations

Now that you know a bit more about basic personality types, let's explore ways in which you can more successfully communicate your needs. Sex and intimacy aren't always easy to discuss, but these basic communication tips can help.

Awareness of Emotional Energy

What is emotional energy? It is the tension in the air that you can cut with a knife; the soft melting feeling when you caress your loved one; or when your bodies are perfectly in tune during a love-making session.

Consider centering yourself before (and during!) the conversation. The breathing exercises in Chapter 16 are a great way to do this. Come to the conversation from a place of peace and desire to make things work for both of you. Then be aware of the energy when you talk. Trust what you feel. If you feel anxious, there's a reason. Don't blame yourself or the other person. You can, however, speak to how you feel and explore that.

Active Listening

People in sales know this technique. It's all about hearing the other person—really listening to them. Not thinking about how you're going to respond, but really hearing their needs, then echoing what you heard them say so you both have the same understanding. For example, "If I understand what you're saying correctly, you'd like to move more slowly because when you feel pressured, you lose desire. Is that right?"

THE BACK AND BEYOND

Avoid the blame game. This is never productive. In fact, it's counter-productive because it makes people defensive. Instead of accusatory statements, such as, "You're selfish in bed," or, "You never want to do it any more," say, "It turns me on when you do more of (your favorite move)," or, "I'd love it if we could be intimate more often, it helps me feel closer to you."

Body Language

Do your words match your body language? If not, body language rules. If you say, "Of course I love you," and roll your eyes at the same time, how do you think that will be interpreted? If you're slumped down on the couch with the game on (even if the sound is off), that's a huge sign that you're not really listening and the conversation isn't very important to you.

Highlight the Good

It's easy to fall into just talking about what's wrong. Talk about what's right in your relationship, too! Review how you got together, when you really knew the person was right for you, and what you value about your relationship now. If there is a particular move you like or want more of in bed, ask your partner. As much as we'd like to think the other person should know us by now, no one is a mind reader. Ask for what you need and want. And definitely let your partner know—in the moment especially—that it feels good!

Don't Fall into the Guilt Trap

You may feel a lot of guilt about having pain and not being the spouse or lover you want to be. In our experience, more men than women say they feel they let their significant other down because their back pain is affecting their sexuality. Men really do have a lot of angst in terms of pleasing their partners (women, take note). Don't let guilt stop you. Instead, have the conversation. There are many ways to rev up and renew your sex life. Clear the air about how you really feel. That in itself can be a turn on for many women!

Romance and Foreplay

With back pain, advance planning may be helpful. The mere anticipation of sex can get the juices flowing for a lot of people. Set a date and time on the calendar. Then create an environment that suits your personalities—music, scented candles, racy movies—whatever works to build the excitement. You may even want to start the night with a hot bath or shower to ease your pain.

Expand your sex and intimacy with new experiences. Massage is a great way to show love and caring. Visit your local adult toy store or shop online for new toys to try. These are especially great when back pain may limit your motion. Let technology help you out! Explore deep kissing and kissing all over. Tickle, nibble, lightly pinch, and tease. Read the *Kama Sutra* (an ancient Indian sex manual) for new ideas. Do a strip tease—guys, you can do this, too! Likewise, champagne with strawberries, red wine with chocolate, or other extravagant sensual delights can make the time more special and enjoyable.

WATCH YOUR BACK

Don't feel the need to rush into intercourse, which can be the most stressful activity on back pain. There are many other pleasure options to try. Be bold. Try something new. See, we told you back pain could improve your sex life!

Positioned for Fun

The cause of your back pain will determine which positions are better for you. This is where that conversation with your doctor will really be important. Knowledge of anatomy is useful here, too. (Check out Chapter 3.) In particular, you want to be aware of the position your back is in. For example, when you arch it, does it hurt more or less? Then choose your position accordingly.

Also, have extra pillows and rolled-up towels ready to use for extra back support. Start slowly and be sure to communicate what's working and what isn't throughout your playtime. When you're done, you might like to have ice or a heating pad handy to conveniently ease any discomfort from the activity.

Side Lying

This is the spooning position. It is a great choice because there is no weight bearing for either person. The person with the back pain can adjust the bend in his or her knees to create a better position for their hips. A pillow placed under the neck and/or to support the waist will help keep the spine aligned and more comfortable during motion. Don't let the shoulder roll forward, as this will twist the upper spine. A pillow under the front knee will also reduce the twist in the lower spine.

Missionary

The person with the back issue is better positioned on the bottom. The position of the knees can vary. The lower back will flex as the knees are pulled farther up, which may lessen lower back pain (again depending on the nature of your pain). The person on top can support his or her body with hands and knees to avoid placing too much weight on the partner. Pillows can be placed under the bottom person's hips and cervical curve of the neck.

Face Down

If your back feels better in a slightly extended or arched position, this might be a good choice. Both partners are lying facing down, one atop the other. A pillow under the bottom person's chest or waist can be helpful. This is not a good position for those with neck issues.

Doggie Style

This is your basic hands and knees position. Again, another good choice if the person with back pain (the one on the bottom) needs to extend the spine. Alternatively, the bottom person can use a chair to support the arms, and the man can enter from a kneeling position.

On a Chair

It's a lap dance! You'll need a chair without arms. Try it in the kitchen or dining room for change of place. The woman sits facing her partner; or facing away works, too. If the man has back pain, a pillow can be placed behind the lumbar spine. A small stool under the feet to prop up the knees a bit helps, too.

THE BACK AND BEYOND

Being in pain typically causes poor posture, being hunched over and miserable. It's hard to feel sexy when your back is on fire and you're hobbling around the bedroom. The internal effects of a body in pain can manifest themselves in your outward appearance, which can really hinder sex drive. That's why taking it slow with romance and sensuality without the pressure of intercourse may be a great way to be intimate.

Pregnancy and Back Pain

Obviously, one of the outgrowths of sex is conception! When that happens, the change a woman's body goes through is nothing short of extraordinary. Back pain is usually a part of the pregnancy package. Here are some common reasons that backs hurt during pregnancy and some suggestions on what you can do about it.

Weight Gain

As the weight of the baby pulls you forward, this will strain your back. Follow your doctor's guidelines for how much weight you really need to gain to support good fetal growth. Many women gain too much weight during pregnancy, which is unhealthy, difficult to lose, and can exacerbate back pain. Don't go on a diet, but do keep your diet healthy.

Exercise is generally fine, although there are limits on what you can do as the weeks go by. Being in the best shape you can before pregnancy will help ease back pain issues, may help childbirth, and will speed recovery, too. Pilates, with its focus on core strength, is really useful before and after. See Chapter 15.

Hormones

A hormone called relaxin loosens ligaments around the pelvic girdle, specifically sacroiliac joints. These ligaments slacken to open up the space for the growing fetus and eventually the delivery process. This laxity can increase the risk of a woman injuring her spine during pregnancy. All of the ligaments in a woman's body tend to relax during pregnancy. Of course, the spine is carrying a lot more weight during this fragile time, so beware!

Of course, you can't and wouldn't want to stop this process, but you can employ many of the same back pain relief techniques in this book such as proper ergonomics for all your activities (see Chapter 18) as well as self-care options such as those in Chapter 5.

The Least You Need to Know

- You don't have to give up sex if you have back pain, but you do have to know more about what you can and can't do physically and emotionally.
- Frank conversation about sex can improve intimacy and pleasure.

- The more you know about your own and your partner's personality profile, the easier it will be to have that sex talk.
- Go slowly, get creative, and be prepared for new adventures in sexuality.

A Pain in the Neck

In This Chapter

- Neck anatomy
- Similarities and differences between neck and back pain
- Factors that make neck pain worse
- Treatments for neck pain

A pain in the neck is like a pain in the rest of your back: the causes vary. It could be due to a garden variety sprain or strain. Also like back injuries, neck injuries tend to go away through time with simple over-the-counter and at-home treatments. But as you undoubtedly know by now, pain—no matter where it is—can also indicate something more serious requiring medical attention.

Because neck pain can accompany back problems, we thought it would be helpful to understand more about your neck, what activities can trigger problems, and the treatment options available to you. Many patients who suffer lower back pain also suffer neck pain because the same disease process can occur in both. Just as hypertension affects your whole body, degenerative disc disease can affect your whole spine, which, of course, includes your neck.

There are also some issues that are unique to your neck. For that, we want to share with you a little neck anatomy. As you'll see, this area of your spine shares similarities with its lower vertebral neighbors, but they also have some important differences.

Neck Anatomy

Your neck is the top of your spine; technically, it is called the cervical spine. Seven vertebrae are in the cervical spine, numbered C1 to C7. C1 is the very top vertebra; C7 the last. C7 can usually be felt easily as it tends to stick out a little bit.

Your neck has a weighty job to do. First, it has to hold up your head, which can weigh on average 8 pounds, and as much as 11 pounds for some! Carry around a bowling ball all day and you'll get some idea of the muscular exertion involved. Like the rest of the spine, the cervical spine also protects your all-important spinal cord.

A problem in the cervical vertebrae can sometimes be the cause of lower back pain. The culprit is often poor head position. With poor posture, your head can cantilever out over your shoulders and cause added strain to your middle and lower back. It's basic body mechanics. When you hold a weight closer to your body (think bicep curls with weights), there's better leverage and joint support. Extend your arms out and away from you and try those same bicep curls again and it'll be much harder and stressful on your joints. Imagine how difficult it would be to hold that bowling ball out in front of you at arm's length. You wouldn't be able to do that for very long without stressing and straining.

> **BODY WISE**
>
> The cervical vertebrae are subject to the same traumas as the rest of the spine, including joint deterioration, bulging discs, and muscle/ligament strain and sprain.

Unlike the vertebrae in the rest of the spine, those in your neck are specially designed to allow your head to move in multiple directions: up and down, side to side, and rotating. This makes the neck a highly sophisticated piece of machinery, but all this flexibility also makes it vulnerable to injury.

The Atlas and the Axis

Two vertebrae in the cervical spine are unlike the others and they have special names. C1 is also known as the Atlas, and, like the Greek god who held up the weight of the world, C1 fits into the top of your skull, holding up your head. The specially shaped bones of the Atlas and the groove in your skull allow you to nod your head up and down like the agreeable person you are.

The Axis, or C2, is specially shaped to allow the rotation that you commonly do when you say "no." Also, there is no intervertebral disc between C1 and C2. These joints notoriously enlarge and become painful in patients with rheumatoid arthritis, but, interestingly, they are not typically affected in osteoarthritis. They are, however, often injured in severe trauma such as motor vehicle accidents.

Discs and Facet Joints

There are cushioning intervertebral discs between the rest of the cervical spine, C2 to C7. Like elsewhere in the spine, these discs can bulge and press on nerves, causing pain. The facet joints cushioned by those discs have many nerve endings, hence the propensity for pain. Cervical facet joints can deteriorate from diseases such as arthritis, or they can be damaged if the head is jerked forward and back such as in whiplash. For more details on discs and facet joints in general, see Chapter 3.

WATCH YOUR BACK

Most patients with degenerative disc disease of the lumbar spine have some degree of the disease in the cervical spine. That's because, as we've mentioned, degenerative disc disease isn't selective—it can affect *any* disc in the spine.

Muscles, Tendons, and Ligaments

The cervical spine is supported by a complex network of ligaments, tendons, and muscles. Because of its high degree of mobility and flexibility, it can be pretty easy to strain the muscles in your neck, which is why posture and ergonomics (see Chapter 18) are especially important.

As you may recall from Chapter 3, tendons attach muscles to bone and ligaments attach bone to bone. There are tendons and ligaments that specifically stabilize the cervical spine. Either or both of these tissues can be traumatized, causing, well, a pain in the neck. Long bands of both of these tissues also extend from the base of the skull all the way down to the tailbone.

These bands of tissue are the targets of *cranio-sacral massage.* They also explain why lower back pain can spread tension to your neck and cause headaches. It's all connected. This interconnection is another reason that patients with neck pain typically have some degree of lower back pain as well. Although we sometimes treat the body as separate parts to be "fixed," remember that the entire system is interrelated.

DEFINITIONS

Cranio-sacral massage is a gentle massage technique that aims to get the spinal cord fluid moving more freely. This fluid runs the length of your spine from your head (cranium) to your tailbone area (sacrum). According to the cranio-sacral theory, when there are blockages, the central nervous system is out of balance. Consequences can include muscle and joint pain as well as emotional disturbances. Massage therapists, physical therapists, and chiropractors are among the main health-care workers that offer the technique. Depending on your insurance policy, it's possible that this treatment by one of these practitioners could be covered.

Cervical Spondylotic Myelopathy

We have talked about a rare and serious condition in the lower back called cauda equina syndrome. When the bundle of nerves in this part of the body is damaged, pain, numbness, weakness, and loss of function in the lower part of the body results.

Cervical spondylotic myelopathy (CSM) is a similarly serious condition that occurs in the upper spine. The spinal canal narrows and the nerves of the spinal cord can get compressed. This can happen for any number of reasons, including degenerative disc disease, bone spurs, or changes in ligaments. Ligaments can either bulge and perhaps thicken to narrow the spinal canal, or can weaken, allowing the bones to slip. Nerve compression in the upper spine affects strength and sensation in arms, trunk, and legs, as well as problems with gait, balance, dexterity, coordination, and fine motor skills. It can even affect breathing, because those nerves travel in the spinal cord at C3 to C5.

Just as with the lower back, some patients are more prone to injury of the cervical spine because they are born with narrower spinal canals. The aging process typically narrows the spinal canal and can lead to cord compression. This myelopathy sometimes requires decompression if patients get weak, fall frequently, or lose function.

The options for decompression are the same as for other parts of the spine. There is anterior (surgical entry from the front of the body) decompression through discectomy and fusion, or posterior (surgical entry from the back of the body) decompression through procedures such as laminectomy or laminoplasty. We explain a bit more about these procedures in a bit.

WATCH YOUR BACK

Cervical spondylotic myelopathy is the most common spinal cord disorder of people 55 years and older.

Radicular Arm Pain

This is like sciatica of the cervical spine. The spinal nerves that exit the cervical vertebra affect the upper half of the body. When the nerves are compressed, it can feel like electrical shocks shooting down your arm and into your hands and fingers. This condition can also cause numbness, weakness, and/or tingling sensations. Usually only one arm is affected, but symptoms can occur in both. Also, turning the head from side to side can be painful with this condition.

The most common cause of radicular arm pain is a bulging disc. Other causes can be bone spurs or, in rare cases, tumor or infection. Electromyography and nerve conduction velocity (EMG/NCV) tests help determine which nerve is affected. See the section on neurological tests in Chapter 12 for details on electromyography.

Most people improve with conservative treatments, including anti-inflammatory and pain meds, and a soft cervical collar. Steroid and nerve-block injections may be used for those cases where the pain persists. If those measures don't work, surgery may be the next logical step.

Surgical Procedures

When all else fails and pain persists, surgery provides relief for many patients. Neck surgery is generally more successful than lower back surgery, for several reasons. First, although the head is relatively heavy, the forces on the neck are overall much lighter than those affecting the lower back.

Second, the neck is much easier to access surgically. Surgeons can expose the neck discs with much less difficulty and tissue trauma, which makes recovery from neck surgery often less painful. Consequently, patient satisfaction is greater. The lower back is complicated by pain generators such as the hips, sacroiliac (SI) joint, and coccyx, as we discussed before. In the neck, the shoulders are far enough away not to cloud the issue.

The available surgical options include the following:

- **Artificial disc:** This procedure replaces a natural disc with an artificial one. Outcomes are more successful in the cervical spine than the lumbar spine. It's also safer because the area is easier to get to if additional surgery is needed. Complications include hoarseness, difficulty swallowing, and persistent pain.

- **Discectomy:** This refers to removing most or the entire intervertebral disc. The surgeon makes an incision on the front of the neck to reach the disc. Fusion accompanies most discectomies because there is very little disc and often most of it has to be removed. Without fusion, there is a higher rate of nerve-root compression when the bones settle into the empty space previously occupied by the disc.

- **Posterior cervical fusion:** In this case, the surgeon goes through the back (posterior) of the neck to fuse two or more vertebrae together. Hardware is used to immobilize the neck. The surgery is most commonly used for neck pain resulting from movement that has caused vertebral bones to become unstable.

- **Cervical laminectomy:** Similar to the lumbar spine surgical technique, a laminectomy is a surgery in which most of the bone called the lamina is removed. This relieves the pressure on the nerves that are causing pain.

- **Cervical laminoplasty:** When there is compression across several levels of the neck, a laminoplasty is a surgical option. The surgeon operates from the back of the neck, but instead of removing the bone (lamina), he or she detaches and elevates the bone on one side to prop open the canal. This increases the space for the spinal cord.

More Distinctions in the Cervical Spine

The cervical spine is different from the rest of the spine in a number of ways:

- Spine disease in this area is a significant source of headaches.

- Degenerative discs in the neck typically result in more bone spurs.

- Because the intervertebral discs are smaller, fusion is more common in the neck.

- Heat and ice treatments are more effective because there is less tissue to heat or cool and you are closer to the muscle and joints that are painful.

- Although the whole body can be thrust forward in a rear-end collision, the neck is more susceptible to whiplash because the head is a heavy weight on a small fulcrum.

- The neck is home to a more complex array of muscles than the rest of the spine.

Neck Pain Causes and Treatments

Most of us have awoken with a crick in our necks or even headaches. Sleeping in an awkward position, like on a train during a long commute home, can do the trick. Also, too many pillows or unsupportive pillows can cause neck pain upon waking.

Specially made cervical pillows mold to the curves in your neck and properly support it during sleep. If you find yourself tucking your hand under your head, or if your head sinks to the bed as soon as you put it on your pillow, it's time to consider a more supportive option.

> **WATCH YOUR BACK**
>
> Propping a phone up to your ear with your shoulder is a sure way to create neck strain. Doing it with a small cell phone can make this even worse. Many hands-free phone devices are available on the market. This alone could eliminate a lot of neck pain. We highly recommend the investment for home and cell phone use.

Computer workers, surgeons, and jewelry repair people are certainly subject to muscular neck strains. Activities such as these encourage your head to jut forward, putting tremendous strain on your muscles, making them tight. The *trapezius* muscle in particular is often the one that tenses up. Making your workspace more ergonomic (see Chapter 18) can help and even eliminate this kind of neck pain.

> **DEFINITIONS**
>
> The **trapezius** is a large muscle that fans out from the back of your skull and extends down to your shoulders. It is the largest of the extensor muscles (those that allow you to move your head backward). When you massage someone and feel little knots under your fingers, it's usually in the trapezius muscle.

Your neck can become sore from overhead lifting or reaching, as when you are painting a ceiling or lifting boxes onto high shelves. Painters, drywall installers, and mural artists are especially vulnerable to neck pain. Massage can help alleviate this kind of pain because it's usually muscular in nature.

WATCH YOUR BACK

Reduce your risk of spinal-cord injury by properly adjusting the height of the head rest in your car. Weekend warriors who play football or drive race cars should use a neck brace.

Another way to relieve neck pain is through some simple stretches. You can simply tilt your ear toward your shoulder (don't raise your shoulder) to get some quick relief. Likewise, if you gently move your chin toward your chest, you'll feel a stretch all the way down between your shoulder blades. If you intertwine your fingers and gently (very gently) pull your head forward, that will increase the stretch.

You should always do neck stretches as isometric exercises. That means you're not trying to see how much you can pull your head forward. You're simply trying to pull against some small resistance to improve muscle tone. Never see how far you can make it go! Small range-of-motion exercises are the key. Rubbernecking to check out a cute girl or guy is not a good idea for someone suffering with neck pain!

The Least You Need to Know

- Many patients who suffer lower back pain also suffer neck pain because the same disease process can occur in both.
- Cervical vertebrae problems can sometimes be the cause of lower back pain. The culprit is often poor head position.
- Because the neck is very flexible, it's easy to strain it. Posture and ergonomics (see Chapter 18) are especially important to reduce neck pain.
- Holding a phone to your ear with your shoulder can lead to neck pain. Use a hands-free device instead.
- When stretching the neck, it's crucial that you do so very gently.

Glossary

acute pain   Pain that comes on suddenly and lasts only a few weeks or less.

addiction   A dependence that occurs when there are adaptive changes in the brain leading to uncontrollable craving for a substance.

alternative medicine   Therapies and practices considered outside of conventional medicine, such as massage and acupuncture. In general, alternative medicine is less invasive (meaning not penetrating the body, such as with surgery), gentler, and based on nature (such as herbal medicine). The practice tends toward holistic practices in that it evaluates the whole person: mind, body, and spirit. Alternative medicines are sometimes used in place of conventional medicine— for example, taking ginger to calm nausea instead of Pepto Bismol.

articulation   The motion that occurs between joints. For example, certain facet joints in the spine allow for up, down, side-to-side, and twisting movements.

bone spurs   Known in medical terminology as osteophytes, a piece of extra bone formed when the body is trying to repair itself. This growth can occur when there is prolonged pressure, rubbing, or stress on bones. When cartilage wears away, a spur may develop. This is not a problem if no other structure is affected, but in the spine, bone spurs might narrow spaces where spinal nerves travel and pinch them.

cartilage   Basically smooth, rubbery connective tissue. Your nose is composed of it as are your ears. Cartilage caps the ends of bones, providing cushion and lubrication enabling bones to move easily. When cartilage wears away, bone grinds on bone, causing pain and deterioration. Osteoarthritis and rheumatoid arthritis are two common diseases that damage joint cartilage. In the spine, facet joints are covered with cartilage.

chronic pain   Pain that, as typically defined, persists for longer than six months.

coccydynia   A painful condition involving swelling around your tailbone. When the ligaments and tendons in this area become inflamed, it hurts to sit. You can also get this pain from a fracture of the coccyx, which can happen if you fall and land on your tailbone.

complementary medicine   Refers to using alternative medicine in combination with conventional practices. These may be patient selected or doctor recommended. For example, using massage and chiropractic methods along with ibuprofen to treat back pain.

connective tissue   Broadly, the various types of tissue that connect and support structures in the body. It's literally everywhere in the body. Collagen, tendons, and even muscles are types of connective tissue. Fascia, a type of connective tissue that lies just under the surface of the skin, can tighten and cause pain in various parts of the body, including the back. Some diseases such as rheumatoid arthritis are considered connective tissues disorders.

conventional medicine   The medical system you're most familiar with, in which medical doctors and other health-care professionals (such as nurses, pharmacists, and therapists) diagnose and treat symptoms and diseases using drugs, therapy, or surgery. It's also called allopathic medicine, mainstream medicine, and Western medicine.

dorsal horn   An area of your spinal cord that receives sensory information from your body, such as touch. The information is processed through two types of cells: transmission cells, which open the pain gate and allow pain signals to travel to the brain; and inhibitory cells, which keep the pain gate closed and help block pain perception.

endorphins Chemicals that the human body produces in response to pain. Drugs made from opiates can stimulate endorphin receptors. They mimic the body's natural pain-killing abilities. Morphine, codeine, opium, and heroin are examples of opiates, drugs derived from the opium poppy.

facet joint The paired joint formed in the back where two vertebrae meet. It is often overlooked as a source of pain.

foramin In anatomical terms, any opening within the body. The plural form is foramina. The term usually refers to a space within or between bones, but it can mean a natural opening within tissues as well.

fractures Cracks in a bone. They can occur in the vertebrae due to disease, overuse, or severe trauma such as a car accident or a fall.

functional training Exercises that support what you do every day, such as standing, picking up children, or climbing up stairs. Well-designed programs build strength and flexibility, which enhance natural movements and coordination between muscles and the nervous system.

integrative medicine A system of medical therapy defined by the National Center for Complementary and Alternative Medicine at the National Institutes of Health as follows: "… integrative medicine combines mainstream medical therapies and CAM therapies for which there is some high-quality scientific evidence of safety and effectiveness." Conventional medical doctors who incorporate these therapies are called integrative.

intervertebral discs The cushion between each vertebra. The disc is composed of two parts: an inner gel-like nucleus, the nucleus pulposus; and a tough outer part, the annulus fibrosus.

intervertebral foramina The holes through which the nerves leave the spine. These holes are the spaces between the upper and lower vertebral bodies. The space is naturally rather narrow. If the space narrows more due to trauma or disease, nerves can get pinched.

joint   The place where two bones come together. In the spine, the joint formed at the meeting of two vertebrae is called a facet joint. Like anywhere in the body, joints can swell and pinch nerves. Many people focus on the discs as a source of back pain although the facet joints are often to blame.

ligaments   Strong fibrous bands that connect bone to bone. Their main job is to stabilize bones, holding them in place. They do, however, have a little flexibility.

neuromuscular reeducation   A therapeutic process for neuro-muscular disorders. Muscles and nerves work together to create movement. Over time, we develop habitual patterns of movement (some good, some not). These are stored in our muscle memory. When there are repetitive poor patterns, trauma, or damage to nerves or muscles, we may need to relearn movements or learn how to do them correctly. That relearning process is called neuromuscu-lar reeducation.

neuropathic pain   Nerve-based pain that reflects trauma, irritation, or chronic changes in nerves. Neuropathic agents are more effective against nerve-related pain.

neuroplasticity   A relatively new concept about how our nervous system participates in memory. When we learn new concepts or experience events, nerves send signals to one another, creating con-nections that can evolve. Through repetition and intensity, lasting connections among neural pathways are made.

nociceptive pain   Pain that originates from tissues in the body (muscle, disc, bone) and is transmitted by the nerves.

peripheral nervous system (PNS)   The collective of the millions of nerves throughout your torso and limbs. PNS nerves convey mes-sages to your central nervous system (CNS), which consists of the brain and spinal cord.

placebo   Inert pills used in clinical trials. They used to be made of sugar, but then they were easily detected as such by the study participants. Now they are a safe but tasteless substance with no biochemical effect. They help determine whether or not a particular substance is effective by comparing outcomes of participants taking placebo versus those who don't.

regenerative medicine   The field of tissue regeneration using stem cells.

stem cells   Cells that can grow into different types of cells—they can become a muscle cell, a red blood cell, or a brain cell. After all, each complex cell in the human body originated from one fertilized egg cell. Experiments have shown that these miraculous cells can also repair or regenerate damaged tissues and restore organ function.

strain/sprain   Injury that results in a pulled, twisted, or torn muscle, tendon, or ligament. A tendon is the end of a muscle that attaches to a bone. A pulled muscle or tendon is called a strain. A ligament attaches bone to bone. When you pull a ligament, it is called a sprain.

surgical loupes   Magnifying lenses worn like glasses. Surgeons commonly use them. These lenses are often custom made to take into account the surgeon's vision.

tendons   Tissue that connects muscles to bones. When a muscle contracts, the signal is concentrated through the tendon, which moves the bone. Tendons are firmly attached to bones. Tendinitis, or inflammation of tendons, can occur even in the spine.

tolerance   The buildup of resistance to the effects of opioids. In other words, your body's metabolism breaks down the current dosage quicker and you need more to get an effect. This is different from addiction but related. Patients develop a tolerance when the current dosage no longer gives them pain relief and they need more.

vertebral column   The spinal column, better known as your backbone. Individual bones are called vertebrae.

Resources

Organizations

American Academy of Medical Acupuncture
Executive Administrator, C. James Dowden
1970 East Grand Avenue, Suite 330
El Segundo, CA 90245
310-364-0193
www.medicalacupuncture.org

This organization promoted the integration of concepts from traditional and modern forms of acupuncture with Western medical training. The site lists medical doctors who perform acupuncture and provides details of the practice.

American Academy of Orthopaedic Surgeons
6300 North River Road
Rosemont, IL 60018-4262
847-823-7186
www.aaos.org

The Academy provides musculoskeletal education to orthopaedic surgeons and has various medical and scientific publications and electronic media materials available.

American Academy of Physical Medicine and Rehabilitation
9700 West Bryn Mawr Avenue, Suite 200
Rosemont, IL 60018
847-737-6000
www.aapmr.org

This organization offers resources on pain management, back and neck treatments, and other physical medicine information.

American Association of Neurological Surgeons
5550 Meadowbrook Drive
Rolling Meadows, IL 60008
847-378-0500 or 1-888-566-AANS (2267)
Fax: 847-378-0600
www.aans.org

The AANS is the organization that speaks for all of neurosurgery. The AANS is dedicated to advancing the specialty of neurological surgery to promote the highest quality of patient care.

American Chiropractic Association
1701 Clarendon Boulevard
Arlington, VA 22209
703-276-8800
www.acatoday.org

The world's largest professional association representing doctors of chiropractic medicine has a patient section that details information about this practice and also has a searchable database of doctors.

American Chronic Pain Association
PO Box 850
Rocklin, CA 95677
1-800-533-3231
www.theacpa.org

This association has information and support for people dealing with chronic pain.

American Medical Association
515 North State Street
Chicago, IL 60654
1-800-621-8335
www.ama-assn.org

On the AMA's site, you can search for medical professionals of all kinds, including those who are not AMA members.

Arthritis Foundation
1330 West Peachtree Street, Suite 100
Atlanta, GA 31193
1-800-283-7800

This voluntary health agency targeted toward consumers has information about all the different types of arthritis, including arthritis of the spine.

Congress of Neurological Surgeons
10 North Martingale Road, Suite 190
Schaumburg, IL 60173
Phone: 847-240-2500
Fax: 847-240-0804
Toll Free: 1-877-517-1CNS
www.cns.org

This organization has details about neurosurgery and a public site where you can search for board-certified neurosurgeons.

Websites

Clinical Trials
clinicaltrials.gov

This website serves as a directory for thousands of worldwide clinical trials in the field of back pain and medicine in general.

Medline Plus
www.nlm.nih.gov/medlineplus

At this National Library of Medicine–produced site, you can find out more about the latest treatments, drugs, and supplements; find out the meanings of words; or view medical videos or illustrations. You can also get links to the latest medical research on your topic or find out about clinical trials on a disease or condition.

National Institute of Health Complementary and Alternative Medicine
nccam.nih.gov

This website provides basic information on complementary and alternative medicine (CAM) including definitions, major types, and resources to learn more.

Neurosurgery Today
www.neurosurgerytoday.org/

The patient side of the AANS, Neurosurgery Today provides patient information on the specialty of neurosurgery and its providers.

SpineBeat
Spinebeat.com

A blog that reviews the latest spine treatments.

SpineUniverse
www.spineuniverse.com

This site has easy-to-search information about back pain, treatments, conditions, back pain exercises, surgery, prevention, and recovery. The site is reviewed by medical doctors, including Dr. Highsmith, the coauthor of this book.

Medical Background Checks

www.abms.org—The American Board of Medical Specialties, the parent organization of the following specialty boards:

> www.abns.org—The American Board of Neurological Surgeons
>
> www.abos.org—The American Board of Orthopedic Surgeons
>
> www.abpmr.org—The American Board of Physical Medicine and Rehabilitation
>
> www.theaba.org—The American Board of Anesthesiology

Physician Reviews

healthgrades.com

vitals.com

These are among several sites where you can check up on a doctor's background, experience, and certifications as well as patient feedback.

Insurance

The Business of Insurance

Learning about health insurance is about as exciting as watching paint dry. Nonetheless, it's valuable to know your rights, what your policy covers, and how to work the system at least somewhat. Research shows that in a 10-year period, American spending on back pain more than doubled. Some $18 billion was spent on physicians, physical therapists, chiropractors, medication, emergency room visits, and other home health-care treatments.

In general, you want your policy to cover at least 80 percent of hospital room and board after your deductible has been met; you also want to be sure the policy has no unreasonable exclusions and an out-of-pocket limit of $3,000 to $5,000 per year.

When it comes to back pain, treatments and policies differ widely. For example, some insurance policies cover complementary and alternative treatments such as massage and chiropractic care; others don't. But that money you spend on over-the-counter meds and treatments may be tax-deductible, depending on how you file your taxes.

Deduct Medical Expenses for Back Pain Treatments

Today, there are a variety of tax-free ways to pay for medical expenses. The most common are flexible spending arrangements (FSAs), health savings accounts (HSAs), and health reimbursement arrangements (HRAs). These accounts are discussed in more detail later in this appendix.

The Internal Revenue Service (IRS) defines a medical expense as the costs of diagnosis, cure, mitigation, treatment, or prevention of disease, and the costs for treatments affecting any part or function of the body. These expenses include payments for legal medical services rendered by physicians, surgeons, dentists, and other medical practitioners. They include the costs of equipment, supplies, and diagnostic devices needed for these purposes. That includes over-the-counter medications and co-payments for doctor visits.

Some expenses not covered by your health insurance, such as eye doctor or dentist visits, are also deductible. But it all depends on how you file your taxes. Search "deductible medical expenses" on the IRS website for more information. Check with your tax preparer as well.

Of course, you'll also always want to consult with your insurance provider before undergoing expensive treatments or assuming what is and isn't deductible as a health expense. Be in the know before you go, to save yourself headaches and hassles down the road.

Policy Basics

All industries love their lingo, and the insurance business is no exception. Notice we said "business." Insurance companies are for-profit businesses. They profit most when they don't have to pay for claims. So it is in your best interest to understand the basics of health insurance.

Insurance policies come in all shapes and sizes. Where you live, whether you smoke, and how old you are constitute a few of the determinants that affect the cost of your policy. Group health insurance is typically offered by employers. If you're self-employed, you may be able to get group rates through unions, professional associations, or other groups.

Health insurance has been in the news a lot lately and it will continue to be as the U.S. government passes new laws about health care. Familiarizing yourself with what's out there will help you make better use of what you have and make more informed choices.

COBRA

The Consolidated Omnibus Budget Reconciliation Act (COBRA) of 1985 tides you over should you lose your job. Under COBRA, employers with 20 or more employees must continue to offer health insurance coverage for 18 months (or sometimes longer) to those who have left the job. You will have to pay the premiums, but that will likely be cheaper than buying a policy on your own because employer-based plans have the advantage of group rates.

Disability Insurance

This, as the name implies, is a policy that will pay benefits if you are too sick to work or become permanently disabled. Payments, policy requirements, and benefits vary widely. Read the fine print carefully; some define disability as the inability to work at *any* job, whereas others say at your *regular* job.

Also, look at when the policy kicks in and how long it lasts. Typically, long-term coverage does not take effect until after 90 days, which won't be useful if you're recovering from back surgery. Short-term disability, however, kicks in right away and provides anywhere from 40 to 60 percent of your base salary for a limited time.

FSA

This stands for flexible spending arrangement. Employers set these up as a benefit for their employees. Employers control and design the plan benefits. Usually both employers and employees contribute to an account. The employee then pulls money from the account for employer-approved health-care expenses. FSAs are generally "use it or lose it" arrangements. That means that the money in the account *is not* carried over from year to year. You use it, or you lose it.

HMO

A health maintenance organization is a type of managed care program where you receive medical care from participating (sometimes called "in-network") providers. Often an HMO requires you to see your primary care doctor before seeing a specialist. When it comes to back pain, you'll want to start with your primary care doc anyway (see Chapter 12).

HSA

A health savings account is set up by an employer or an individual. These accounts often come with debit cards, which are handy for over-the-counter medical products as well as for co-payments. The account allows you to save money toward medical expenses on a tax-free basis. Unlike with FSAs, any balance remaining at the end of the year "rolls over" to the next year. Also, you do not have to have an HSA to deduct IRS-approved medical expenses. It can make the accounting a bit easier, however.

High-Risk Pool

If you can't get health insurance from other sources because of a serious illness, high-risk pools can help. The new health-care law provides money to states to either administer the program themselves (according to federal rules) or agree to let the Federal Department of Health and Human Services run it. Some states already have their own high-risk pool in place. Premiums and coverages vary.

Indemnity

Unlike an HMO, with this type of health insurance you can use any doctor or hospital for medical care. The provider sends the bill to the insurance company, which pays a portion of it. The advantage of this type of plan is that it often covers medical expenses that other types of plans do not. The disadvantage may be higher monthly premiums.

Long-Term Care

This type of policy pays for all or part of the cost of home health-care services or care in a nursing home or assisted living facility.

Medicare and Medicare Supplemental Insurance (Medigap)

Medicare is a federal insurance program that provides health-care coverage to individuals age 65 and older and certain disabled people. Medigap is health insurance sold by private insurance companies to fill the "gaps" in Medicare, paying some of the health-care costs that the original Medicare plan doesn't cover. Insurance companies can only sell you a "standardized" Medigap policy, which must all have specific benefits so you can easily compare them.

Medicaid

This federal program provides health care for low-income people. Although it is a federal program, it is run by states and features vary by state.

PPO and PSO

A preferred provider organization (PPO) is a type of managed care plan. Compared to an HMO, a PPO provides more flexibility in choosing physicians and other providers. You can see both participating and nonparticipating providers, but your out-of-pocket expenses will be lower if you see only plan providers.

Similarly, a point-of-service (PSO) plan is also a type of managed care plan. With a PSO, primary care physicians coordinate patient care, but there is more flexibility in choosing doctors and hospitals than in an HMO.

Common Terms to Know

There's a lot to know about your own individual policy. These are a few of the basics that apply to most plans. Knowing these will help you better use your health-care benefits.

Co-Pay

This is the flat fee you pay when you visit a doctor. Your insurance covers the rest.

Deductible

This is the annual amount you must pay before your insurance policy kicks in. The higher the deductible, the lower your monthly premiums.

Exclusions and/or Limitations

This is what your insurance policy does not cover. Exclusions and limitations must be clearly spelled out in plan literature, but there can still be a lot of confusion over what is and isn't covered. If you're unsure, talk to your agent or insurance representative before you assume anything either way.

Out-of-Pocket

This is the amount you pay in addition to your monthly premiums. This can include your annual deductible and co-payments. Plans have a ceiling on the annual amount you'd have to pay, which is expressed as out-of-pocket maximum. A survey showed that back pain sufferers paid about 17 percent out of pocket on back pain care expenses, private health insurance paid 45 percent, Medicare 23 percent, and other sources, including workers' compensation, paid 15 percent.

Premium

This is what you have to pay to belong to a health plan. It's usually a monthly payment. If you have employer-sponsored health insurance, your share of premiums usually is deducted from your pay.

Emergency Care

Does your policy include emergency room visits? And are there any requirements? Some health plans require notification within 24 hours of going to an emergency room, or the expenses will not be covered. Some require you to call your primary care physician first, unless the condition is life threatening. Exactly how does your plan define "life threatening"? Severe sciatica may be debilitating, but it's generally not life threatening; however, if cauda equina is suspected, that's another matter. Depending on your plan, your choice of hospital may be limited. Understand your policy clearly before making assumptions.

Preexisting Conditions

The health-care reform bill that passed in 2010 outlawed the denial of insurance based on preexisting conditions. The policy took effect for children in September 2010, but it won't become a requirement for adults until 2014. In the meantime, high-risk pools (see the section "High-Risk Pool" earlier in the chapter) can help those who have difficulty obtaining insurance.

Workers' Compensation and Back Pain

This is a form of social insurance that provides injured workers with medical care, income (or a percentage of income), and survivor benefits in cases of fatalities. Note, however, that the worker who claims workers' comp benefits waives the right to sue his or her employer.

Laws and Disputes

There are specific laws protecting your right to health benefits when you lose coverage or change jobs. In particular, the following references from the U.S. Department of Labor can help.

The Employee Retirement Income Security Act (ERISA)

This act offers protection for individuals enrolled in retirement, health, and other benefit plans sponsored by private-sector employers, and provides rights to information and a grievance and appeals process for participants to get benefits from their plans.

The Health Insurance Portability and Accountability Act

Better known as HIPAA, this act includes protections for millions of working Americans and their families who have preexisting medical conditions, prohibits discrimination in health-care coverage, and guarantees issuance of individual policies for certain eligible individuals.

In addition, the following brochures can help. Call Employment Benefits and Security Administration (EBSA) toll-free at 1-866-444-EBSA (3272) to get hard copies or view them on the web at www.dol.gov/ebsa.

- *Your Health Plan and HIPAA: Making the Law Work for You*

- *An Employee's Guide to Health Benefits Under COBRA*

- *Filing a Claim for Your Health or Disability Benefits*

- *Retirement and Health Care Coverage: Questions and Answers for Dislocated Workers*

- *Can the Retiree Health Benefits Provided by Your Employer Be Cut?*

- *Life Changes Require Health Choices: Know Your Benefit Options*

- *Work Changes Require Health Choices: Protect Your Rights*

Frequently Asked Questions

We live in an instant-gratification world, so here we'll just cut to the chase to give you quick answers to the most frequently asked questions about back pain. We reference chapters where you can get more details on a particular subject.

Why is back pain so prevalent?

In short, genetics and "wear and tear" are the main reasons that so many people experience back pain at some point in their lives. Either we're not moving enough or we're moving incorrectly. Some people are genetically predisposed to having back issues, but most suffer because of a mechanical malfunction—a strained muscle, for example. A number of physical risk factors can contribute to back problems:

- Heavy physical work
- Lifting and forceful movements
- Bending and twisting
- Whole-body vibration
- Static work postures

Stress and psychological issues can also contribute to back pain. For more on this subject, see Chapters 1 and 4.

Why is it so hard to diagnose?

The human body is complicated, to say the least. And everyone's body is unique. Think about all the things that can go wrong with your computer and you can appreciate why diagnosing the human machine can be so challenging. There are three types of cartilage alone in the human spine. Pain generators include bones, muscles, ligaments, tendons, facet joints, facet capsules, discs, and nerves. See Chapter 4 for more on diagnostics and Chapter 3 for information about anatomy.

Why is it so hard to cure?

The short answer, again, is that it's complicated. The interaction of all of these multiple components is exponentially more complex. Seldom is there a problem in just one focal point. Most back pain is the result of the entire system being askew. The good news is that most back pain does get better in time, and there are lots of ways for you to help yourself feel better (see Chapter 5).

How long does it take a disc to repair?

It takes several months because the disc is the largest organ in the body with no blood supply. That means it slowly absorbs the nutrients it needs from surrounding tissue. Disc bulges are not uncommon. We can have them and never experience back pain if the bulge is not disturbing the bones or nerves. However, a torn or degenerated disc can remain injured for a lifetime. Even when a disc heals, it is never as strong as it was. Just like a car that has been in an accident, a disc that is damaged is never quite the same again.

Do chiropractic treatments really work?

Depending on what's wrong with your back, yes, the treatments can help. The idea behind chiropractic treatments is to realign your spine. Vertebral bones can slightly shift out of place for a number of reasons, including poor posture, repetitive physical stress, or injury. Chiropractors manually adjust the spine to move the bones back where they belong.

However, avoid chiropractic treatments if you have any disease that weakens bones, such as osteoporosis, rheumatoid arthritis, or bone cancer. See Chapter 7 for more on this and other complementary and alternative treatments.

How long do epidural injections last? And how do they work?

Patients might feel better right away because of the numbing effect of the anesthetic, but it usually takes several days to feel the full effect of an epidural steroid. Injections may last several months, and patients generally require another dose or two before the natural healing process of the body has taken place. Other times, the injection may last only a few days.

The injection works by reducing pain and inflammation. It does not repair the disc, but buys time while the disc heals.

What does it mean to "shave" a disc?

This is a lay term that really is a misnomer. Surgeons never really shave a disc; they simply remove the bulging portion.

How much is removed in a discectomy?

This varies. Sometimes surgeons simply remove the free fragment (ruptured portion). Other times, a larger portion of the bulge is removed along with any loose tissue that may reherniate. The amount of material removed may only be 5 percent or could be 80 percent. Removing it all makes the disc unstable and collapses, leaving the spine with bone on bone. Obviously, we want to avoid this.

How can a disc reherniate if I have already had a discectomy?

Surgeons typically leave any disc material they can in order to provide cushion. Sometimes a piece of disc that was intact previously can herniate in the same manner as the previous one did. Surgeons remove the entire disc only if they are performing a fusion.

How long does it take nerve damage to repair?

Nerves can repair to some degree, but not always completely. You've witnessed it when you have cut your finger and develop a numb spot that goes away after a few weeks. It can take several months, even up to a year or so in some cases. Nerves can be damaged from the initial injury, prolonged pressure, or surgical complications. Some "nerve damage" is simply leftover problems from the nerve not healing completely.

Why aren't artificial discs as popular as hip and knee replacements?

The hip and knee are fairly simple joints compared to the spine. The spine allows compression (shock absorption), stretching, flexion/

extension, lateral bending, twisting/rotation, and sliding movements. Each level of the spine has a disc and two paired facet joints. Often the disease process is found in all three. Simply replacing the disc will allow more motion at that level, including more motion in the facets, which may be causing the pain in the first place.

I heard spinal fusions are dangerous and rarely really needed.

Although fusions are quite invasive, they can be lifesavers for those whose joints are totally deteriorated and whose bone spurs obstruct nerve passages. Fusion is actually what the body does naturally in response to some traumatic conditions. Some people may find their mobility is actually better after fusion because they are no longer in pain.

Typically fusion is most effective for patients with only a few levels of disease who have instability and/or significant changes on MRI. Read Chapter 9 for more on fusions and other surgical procedures.

It takes forever for the FDA to approve new procedures. Is it really that risky to get treatment out of the country?

It can be. Complications can occur and local physicians are reluctant to pick up where foreign physicians have left off. Many of the experimental treatments are just that—experimental, often with less rigid study designs and shorter follow-up than more conservative regulatory agencies such as the FDA require. Also, don't expect your insurance to cover such treatment. You might be better off looking for clinical trials in this country. See Chapter 10 for more.

I admit it, I'm lazy. Does exercise really make a difference?

In a word, yes. It helps maintain a healthy spine and it's vital for rehabbing from back pain and injuries. For the majority of people who have common strain/sprain back pain, exercise will help relieve pain and reduce the chances of its reoccurrence.

Of course, exercise is no guarantee that your back will never hurt. Sometimes a wrong move or too much exercise can actually cause a problem. But the bottom line is that if you want to feel good in your body, you need to exercise your body. See Chapters 14 through 17 for exercises to keep your back healthy.

Do special mattresses help?

They can. What you don't want to do is sleep on a saggy mattress. You want one that supports your spine's natural curves. Ergonomics modifies an environment to align with your body. That's as true for mattresses as it for aligning computers and car seats. See Chapter 18 to learn more.

I feel really nervous about having sex. Is it OK to do it?

Whether you have the back issue or your partner does, one of the easiest ways to get started on your journey back to sexual intimacy is to talk about it. We get you started in Chapter 19 and offer you some back-friendly ways to get in the mood and play!

Index

A

abdominal muscles, 34-35, 182
  strengthening, 171
Accreditation Commission for
  Acupuncture and Oriental
  Medicine (ACAOM), 165
acetaminophen, 48, 68
acupressure, 96-97
acupuncture, 96-97, 105
acupuncturists, 159
acute back pain, 9
  versus chronic back pain, 14
aerobic exercise, 171, 211-214
alternative medicine, 11, 162
  CAM (complementary and
    alternative medicine), 93-101,
    157-158, 162
  herbalists, 164-165
  homeopaths, 164
  naturopaths, 162-163
  TCM (traditional Chinese
    medicine), 165
alternative nostril breathing,
  yoga, 195
American Academy of Medical
  Acupuncture, 138
American Academy of
  Neurological Surgeons, 138
American Academy of
  Orthopedic Surgeons, 122, 138

American Academy of Physician
  Acupuncturists (AAPA), 159
American Association of
  Neurological Surgeons, 122
American Board of Medical
  Specialties (ABMS), 136
American Chiropractic
  Association, 138
American College of Sports
  Medicine (ACSM), 206
American Council on Exercise
  (ACE), 206
American Herbalists Guild, 165
American Massage Therapy
  Association, 138
American Medical Association
  (AMA), 138
American Osteopathic
  Association, 138
American Physical Therapy
  Association, 138
ankylosing spondylitis, 51-52
annulus fibrosus, 31, 47
anterior longitudinal ligament,
  34
anti-inflammatory drugs
  (NSAIDs), 48
anti-inflammatory medications,
  84-85
antidepressants, 105
antigravity chairs, 77
arm pain, radicular, 243-244

F

G

H

I

O

P

U–V

W–X–Y–Z